THE *ESSENTIAL*
PANDEMIC
SURVIVAL GUIDE

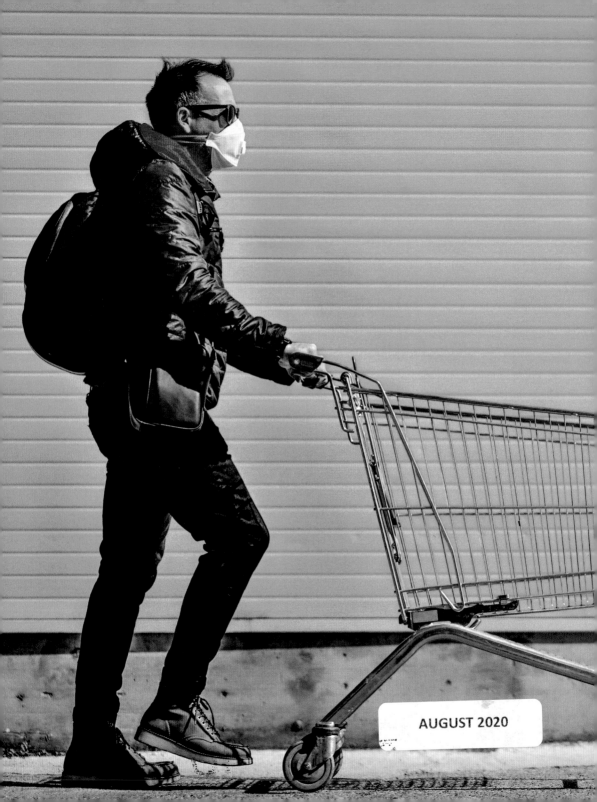

AUGUST 2020

THE *ESSENTIAL*
PANDEMIC
SURVIVAL GUIDE

TIM MACWELCH

JOSEPH PRED

weldon**owen**

CONTENTS

CHAPTER 5: PLAN AHEAD

CHAPTER 6: GET OFF THE GRID

CHAPTER 7: EXTREME OUTCOMES

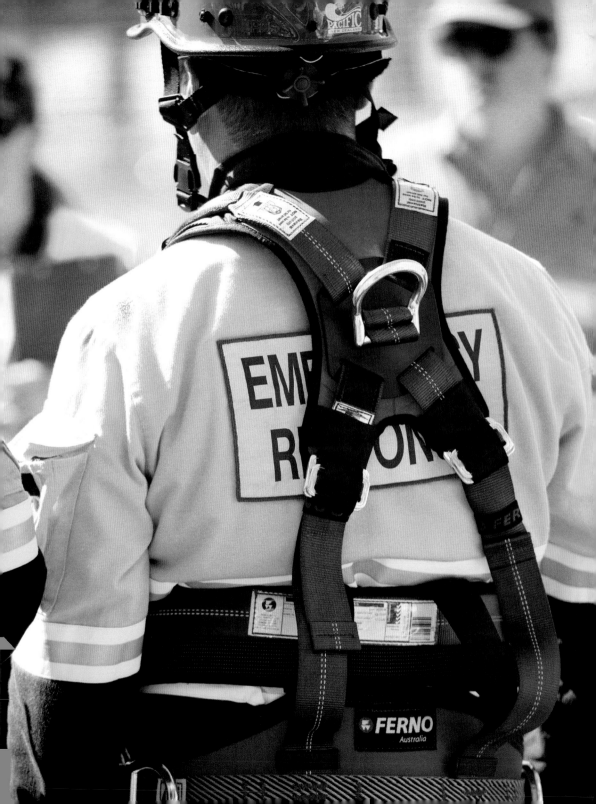

STAY SAFE & HEALTHY

As an Emergency and Risk Manager with over twenty years experience, you could say I'm a disaster geek. That's because for me each phase of the disaster planning cycle is very important, be it preparing, mitigating, responding, or recovery. While everyone can connect with the exciting aspects of responding to an emergency of the sirens blaring, running bravely into the danger zone variety, few realize that what makes such heroics possible starts with the parts that might actually seem as quite boring. Planning, checklists, training and logistics are all invisible when large incidents happen and you see people coming to the rescue, but that's honestly what gets you to the finish line. Without this essential planning, your chances of making it even past the starting line are slim. While nothing can truly stop the devastation of a pandemic, what you do in advance can make the inevitable recovery period much easier for you and your family. After all, this is going to be stressful enough as it is without also having to buy supplies, figure out all the details, and learn how to keep yourself safe in the middle of a pandemic.

When first presented with the idea of collaborating with Tim I didn't hesitate and instantly said I was on board with co-authoring this book with him. From my Emergency and Risk Management experience you might wonder how an expert in primitive technology and outdoor survival swould mesh with my first responder perspective. But actually, Tim's knowledge and experience is the perfect counterbalance. While I've seen plenty of emergency preparedness books written either by a survival pro or an emergency responder, each has their own unique angle on how to survive disasters, and never had I seen one that combined both perspectives into one volume. Based on Tim's previous writing I knew we would bring a point of view to this book that would complement each other's strengths.

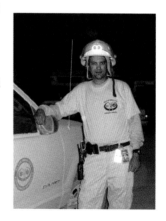

It wasn't until the 2020 Coronavirus pandemic that I realized the lack of disaster preparedness books specifically focused on infectious disease. While most disasters are regional in scale, pandemics are global and include an avalanche of information from the media and the internet. It's easy to get overwhelmed. Reading this handbook will give you the skills to plan and the confidence to be resilient enough to survive future pandemics.

JOSEPH PRED
Founder, Mutual Aid Risk & Safety

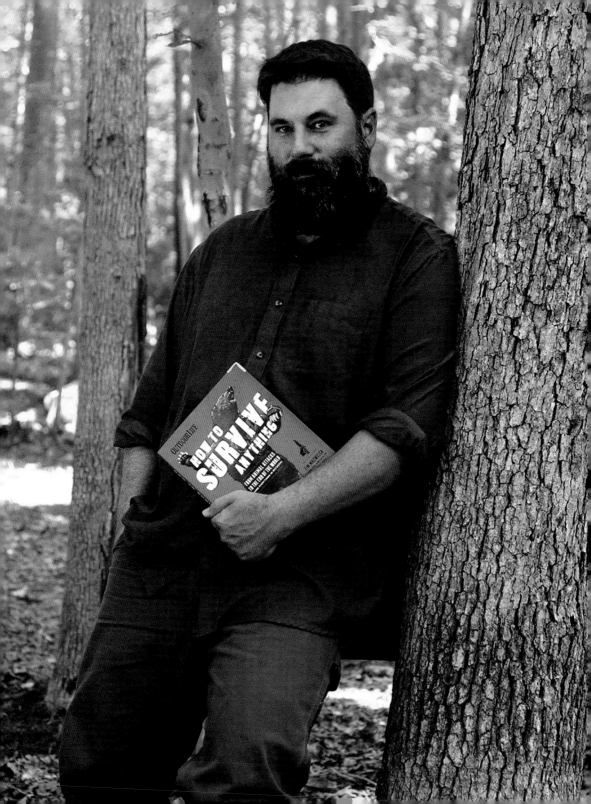

SURVIVE A PANDEMIC

I've been a survival instructor for more than two decades, and I can tell you from experience that there's nothing easy about survival in any type of emergency scenario. But if we look at history, survival was our day job as early humans. In ancient times, we scrambled to protect ourselves from threats and we struggled to acquire the supplies to help us last one more day. In a modern crisis, it can feel like we have returned to that stressful hand-to-mouth way of life. Our shelters, garb, and technology are different, but our needs and vulnerabilities haven't changed in tens of thousands of years. We need the same things we have always needed, and we can be harmed in the same ways we've faced forever. Our "caves" may be air-conditioned now, but we still hide in them to protect ourselves from the threats of the day (like viruses and desperate people). As we make "supply runs" to the store in the midst of disease, these hunting and gathering trips can feel like an expedition to some hostile landscape. While this all sounds rough, there is a bright side: We can find comfort in continuity. Our ancestors made it through plague after plague, for thousands of years and they did it with fewer resources and less knowledge than we possess today. If they endured, we can too. It's just going to take some hard work.

Getting sick and fighting over the last roll of toilet paper aren't the only hardships we face in a pandemic. We may lose our jobs due to the injured economy or lose a relationship due to the stress and strain of the situation. Pandemics are like a sucker punch, coming out of nowhere and striking us by surprise. That's bad enough, but then the crisis keeps tossing surprises at us. In times like these, it's going to take both skills and knowledge to keep you from becoming victim and turn you into a survivor. By cultivating your inherent traits of adaptability and tenacity, you can endure when things get tough. By planning ahead and learning new skills, you make yourself (and your household) more resilient and better able to adapt to change. In short, you are hard-wired for survival, and we are here to help you make the most of that.

In this book, my co-author Joseph and I are going to show you how to prepare for the worst, share methods to manage your own survival, help you plan how to take care of your loved ones and friends, and provide ways to face a crisis that has dogged humanity for thousands of years—the scenario of a deadly epidemic. Don't worry, it's not all doom and gloom. Sometimes, it takes a crisis to peel away the distractions and noise of our busy lives, to remind us the things that matter the most to us.

TIM MACWELCH
Founder, Advanced Survival Training

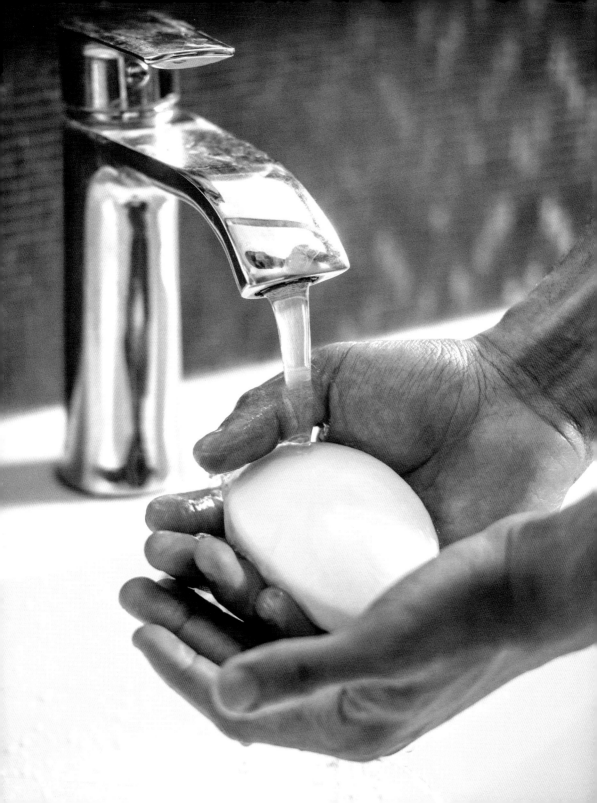

THE BASICS

There are a wide range of skills and tips in this book, from quick survival solutions to more elaborate plans, from everyday needs to worst-case scenarios. Before you jump ahead, it's smart to build a foundation of knowledge.

Sometimes, the simplest things can make the biggest difference. Before we show you how to gear up for emergencies or help you "head for the hills" to escape, you'll need to lay the groundwork for pandemic safety. Nothing can be built up without a solid foundation.

KNOW WHAT'S GOING ON In a pandemic, it often feels as though the guidelines and projected outcomes are changing every day—and often, that's because they are. In this chapter, we give you the basic information you need to know about the novel coronavirus, as well as best-practice tactics for any outbreak or epidemic.

KEEP IT CLEAN Washing your hands really does work to prevent the spread of disease and this simple practice might just save your life, but your hands aren't the only thing to keep clean. Learn to harness you inner "clean freak" by disinfecting items that come from the outside and prevent cross-contamination in your home.

AVOID THE SCAMS Tough times can bring out the best in people, as communities rally to help each other. Unfortunately, they can also bring out the worst. Bogus "cures" that do more harm than good, phishing scams, and identity thievery are just a few of the hazards we face—above and beyond the plague at our doorsteps.

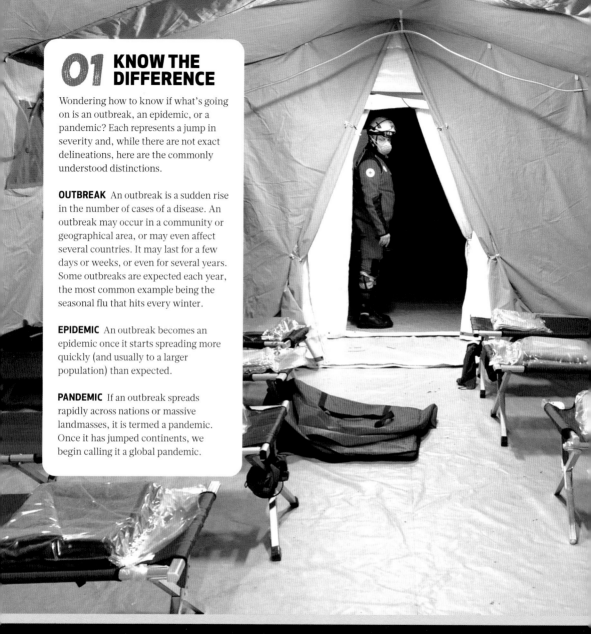

01 KNOW THE DIFFERENCE

Wondering how to know if what's going on is an outbreak, an epidemic, or a pandemic? Each represents a jump in severity and, while there are not exact delineations, here are the commonly understood distinctions.

OUTBREAK An outbreak is a sudden rise in the number of cases of a disease. An outbreak may occur in a community or geographical area, or may even affect several countries. It may last for a few days or weeks, or even for several years. Some outbreaks are expected each year, the most common example being the seasonal flu that hits every winter.

EPIDEMIC An outbreak becomes an epidemic once it starts spreading more quickly (and usually to a larger population) than expected.

PANDEMIC If an outbreak spreads rapidly across nations or massive landmasses, it is termed a pandemic. Once it has jumped continents, we begin calling it a global pandemic.

02 KNOW ABOUT ARDS

People who end up in intensive care due to Covid-19 often suffer from acute respiratory distress syndrome, or ARDS, which impairs the lungs' ability to exchange oxygen and carbon dioxide. This can result in organ failure, brain damage, abnormal heart rhythms, and other serious conditions. The signs and symptoms of ARDS can begin

within hours to days of infection; treatment uses a ventilator. Globally, ARDS affects more than 3 million people a year, as it can also occur from conditions such as pneumonia, sepsis, severe burns, and smoke inhalation. ARDS has a mortality rate of approximately 40% and even for those who survive, a decreased quality of life is sadly common.

03 IF YOU READ NOTHING ELSE

While the specifics of any outbreak will keep changing and evolving as the virus does, there are some basic practices that are almost always appropriate.

- ☐ **WASH YOUR HANDS** If you're feel like you're washing your hands too often and for too long, you're probably doing it just enough.

- ☐ **USE HAND SANITIZER** If you can't wash your hands with soap and water, then this is the next best thing.

- ☐ **WEAR A MASK** A cloth or dust mask works fine to protect others from droplet transmission.

- ☐ **COVER YOUR MOUTH** Cough or sneeze into the crook of your arm if you don't have a tissue.

- ☐ **DON'T TOUCH YOUR FACE** Wearing a face mask helps keep your hands off your nose and mouth, but remember to not touch your eyes either, as an infection get into your system that way as well.

- ☐ **WEAR SAFETY GLASSES** To protect your eyes from airborne pathogens and keep you from touching your eyes.

- ☐ **KEEP AWAY** Consider 6 feet (2 m) as a minimum standard to avoid aerosol transmission from people nearby, even if they have no symptoms.

- ☐ **STAY HOME** Feeling sick? Stay home to avoid infecting others and seek medical attention if you feel worse.

- ☐ **PROTECT OTHERS** If someone in your household is sick, assume you also are contagious.

- ☐ **SHELTER IN PLACE** Remaining at home is the safest way to avoid exposure.

- ☐ **WIPE IT DOWN** Disinfect doorknobs, alarm keypads, or frequently touched surfaces, especially anything else you touch when first entering your home.

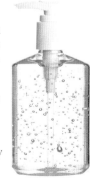

- ☐ **RINSE OFF** If you must go anywhere, change clothes and shower as soon as you get home.

- ☐ **PRACTICE SELF CARE** Eating well, sleeping well, and exercising regularly can bolster your immune system.

04 FOCUS ON CORONAVIRUS

Coronaviruses cause diseases in humans, mammals, and birds; when one crosses between species, it can go from being be mild in the original species to deadly in others. Often these start as a novel CoronaVirus (nCoV), the term for a medically significant new coronavirus . In humans the viruses cause respiratory tract infections which can range from mild to lethal. It is estimated about 15% of common colds in humans are caused by coronaviruses. In recent decades, several zoonotic coronaviruses (those that began with an animal strain and crossed over to us) have caused series outbreaks.

SARS The severe acute respiratory syndrome coronavirus (SARS-CoV) led to the 2002-2004 SARS outbreak. Over 8,000 people from 29 different countries and territories were infected, and at least 774 died worldwide with a fatality rate of 9.2%. SARS is known to have crossed over from to humans either directly from horseshoe bats or by way of wild civet meat sold at a local market in Guangdong, China.

MERS The first outbreak of Middle East respiratory syndrome-related coronavirus (MERS-CoV), was the 2012 MERS outbreak in the Middle East, followed by the 2015 MERS outbreak in South Korea and the 2018 MERS outbreak centered in Saudi Arabia. MERS has been genetically linked to Camels and Egyptian tomb bats as the zoonotic source of human infection. Globally MERS patients were reported in over 25 countries, with almost 2500 cases worldwide and over 850 deaths reported, giving it a fatality rate of 36%.

COVID-19 The Coronavirus 2 (SARS-CoV-2), the cause of the global COVID-19 pandemic, is a strain of the original SARS virus. The first known patient was infected in Wuhan, the capital of China's Hubei province, in November 2019. The virus subsequently spread to all provinces of China and to more than 150 other countries worldwide. Most people with COVID-19 recovered. For those who do not, the time from development of symptoms to death has been between 6 and 41 days, with an average 14 days. From a global perspective, the infection fatality rate is estimated to be up to 0.4%. However, of those who are admitted the hospital, the fatality rate is much higher, with a death to case ratio of approximately 6.2% at the time of writing.

05 UNDERSTAND THE TERMINOLOGY

With the news cycle being faster than ever, it's important to recognize that sometimes the media doesn't use scientific or medical terms correctly and that can cause confusion. To be well informed, you'll do well to know the basic terminology of pandemics.

CLUSTER A collection of cases occurring in the same place at the same time. If clusters are of sufficient size and severity, they may be upgraded to an outbreak.

COMMUNITY TRANSMISSION The term for cases of infection in persons who haven't traveled recently and have no connection to a known case. Also called "community spread."

CONTACT TRACING The practice of identifying and locating people who have been exposed to a known contagious person. They are then either asked to self-quarantine or brought in for observation in order to prevent transmission.

CONTAGIOUS Transmissible by direct or indirect contact with an infected person or thing. For example, the coronavirus is both contagious and infectious. Anything that is contagious is also infectious, but the reverse is not necessarily true.

DROPLET TRANSMISSION How a contagious disease is spread when it involves relatively large, short-range respiratory droplets produced by sneezing, coughing, or talking. Also called "aerosol transmission."

EPIDEMIC The rapid spread of disease to a large number of people across a very large area within a short period of time.

FLATTEN THE CURVE This refers to the goal of slowing a virus's spread to reduce the peak number of cases. This does not necessarily decrease the total number of cases; it just spreads them out over a longer period so that hospitals can cope with the number of patients at any given time rather than being overwhelmed.

HERD IMMUNITY A form of community protection from a disease that occurs when a large percentage has become immune, whether through previous infections or vaccination, thereby providing some measure of protection for individuals who are not yet immune.

INFECTIOUS Producing, capable of producing, or containing pathogens which can be transmitted. For example, food poisoning is infectious, but it is not contagious.

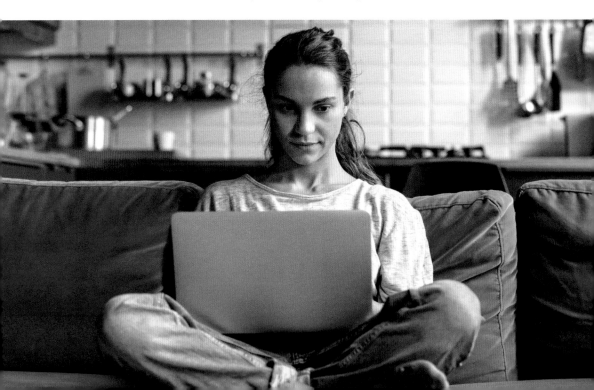

ISOLATION Methods used to separate patients infected with a communicable disease to isolate them from healthy persons, usually in a healthcare setting.

LOCKDOWN A government order preventing people from entering or leaving a specific area without special permission or performing essential functions.

OUTBREAK A sudden rise in the number of cases of a disease in a specific region.

PANDEMIC An epidemic that crosses international boundaries, affecting people on a multiple continents.

PPE This stands for "Personal Protective Equipment," the specialized clothing and equipment such as masks and hazmat suits used as a safeguard against physical, chemical, or biological hazards.

QUARANTINE Separating and restricting the movement of people exposed (or potentially exposed) to a contagious disease.

R0=x Pronounced "R-naught," an estimate of the average number of new cases of a disease that each infected person generates. R0 estimates for the virus that causes COVID-19 are R0=~2-3, which is slightly higher than that for seasonal flu (R0=~1.2-1.3), but far lower than more contagious diseases such as measles (R0=~12-18).

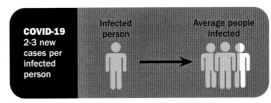

COVID-19 2-3 new cases per infected person — Infected person → Average people infected

SHELTER IN PLACE A directive issued by local, state or national government in which residents are either asked or ordered to remain at their place of residence, except to conduct essential activities.

SOCIAL DISTANCING Measures taken to reduce person-to-person contact in order to stop or slow down the spread of a contagious disease.

ZOONOSIS The process by which an infectious disease caused by a pathogen jumps from n animals to humans. More than two-thirds of human viruses are thought to be zoonotic.

06 BEWARE THE SUPER SPREADER

What is a "super spreader"? This is a person who infects a disproportionately high number of people, compared to number of people infected by the average sick person. In some of the cases of super-spreading, these infected people conform to the 20/80 rule. This means that roughly 20% of infected individuals cause up to 80% of the illness transmissions. A frightening proposition, if the disease is lethal. Perhaps the best known super spreader was Mary Mallon, also known as Typhoid Mary. Mallon was a cook for a number of different families in New York City. She was an asymptomatic carrier of typhoid fever, a potentially deadly disease caused by the bacteria *Salmonella typhi*. Mallon infected 51 people between 1902 to 1909. Three of those infected died from the illness. She was eventually placed under involuntarily quarantine (locked up) by public health authorities at Brothers Island in New York, until her death in 1938. If you don't have strong COVID-19 symptoms, but everyone around you gets sick after your close contact—you might be a super spreader. All the more reason for everyone to stay the hell at home.

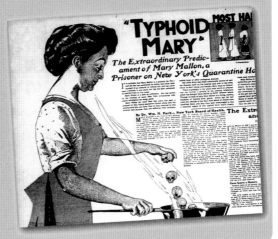

07 WASH LIKE A SURGEON

Nothing fights germs like frequent and thorough hand washing. Even though we've been washing our hands without help since childhood, it's smart to consider the hand-washing details that doctors employ. Short fingernails, good washing technique, warm water, and ample soap might just stop the next pandemic before it starts.

STEP 1 Turn on the warm water and wet your hands.

STEP 2 Apply soap to the palms and backs of your hands.

STEP 3 Rub your soapy palms together.

STEP 4 Rub your palm on the back of your hand, threading the fingers of your top hand between your lower fingers.

STEP 5 Rub your palms together, interlacing your fingers and scrubbing them.

STEP 6 Bend your fingers under, face your hands palm to palm, and scrub your fingernails together.

STEP 7 Wash each thumb by using the opposite hand to twist it.

STEP 8 Using your fingernails, scrub the palm of each hand in a circular motion.

STEP 9 Rinse both hands with warm water.

STEP 10 Dry your hands with a disposable paper towel.

STEP 11 Turn off the water, using the paper towel as a barrier to the faucet handle.

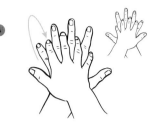

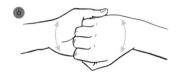

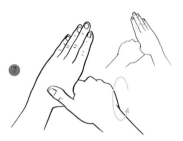

08 SING A 20-SECOND SONG

By this point, everyone (hopefully) knows that you should be washing your hands for at least 20 seconds, or as long as it takes for you to sing "Happy Birthday" twice. But man is that tune getting tired! Here are some other options for your hand-washing pleasure.

- One full chorus of Prince's "Raspberry Beret."
- Lady Macbeth's "Out Damn Spot" monologue from, duh, *Macbeth*.
- The chorus to Beyoncé's "Love on Top." Belt it out like the Queen Bey of the washroom.
- The chorus to Dolly Parton's "Jolene," with as much slow-mo emotion as you can muster.
- "Baby Shark" at least twice through the entire Shark family.

- Three times through the rousing "We Will Rock You" chorus from Queen's song of the same name. Style points if you shout-sing "We will, we will, wash you! (Wash you!)" to your hands.
- More into reality TV? *E News* suggests a heartfelt rendition of Peter's mom's viral plea from *The Bachelor*: "Bud, Hannah Ann loves you with all of her heart. Don't let her go. Don't let her go. Bring her home to us."

09 HELP KIDS WASH UP

To be sure kids wash long enough, help them time a 20-second rhyme they'll remember, or try this version of the old standard: "Twinkle, twinkle little star. Look how clean my two hands are. Around my wrists, now twist that thumb, lace my fingers, almost done. Twinkle, twinkle little star. Look how clean my two hands are."

10 BE SAFE ABOUT GROCERY SHOPPING

We don't know how you feel about going to get groceries. Some people have always hated food shopping. For the homemaker types, it wasn't so bad in former times. You'd push the cart through the store (bare handed!) and plan some meals that the family would like. You might buy a few days worth of food, bring the bags home and plop them right on the countertop where the food is prepared.

Today, things are not so easy. At some point, the groceries in your kitchen are going to dwindle and you're going to have to resupply. This means a trip to the grocery store, and possible exposure to the coronavirus. Even if you wear gloves and a mask in the store, many people have touched your food packages, which you have touched after touching the shopping cart handle.

And don't even remind us about the poor, beleaguered checkout worker, who has touched everything that has been handled by customers (both healthy and sick) and then touched each and every item you buy. This is why you need to set up a decontamination station at home. Here's how.

STEP 1 Pick a cleaning station. This should *not* be your kitchen table (where you eat the food) or your kitchen counter (where you prep it). We know folks who use a plastic table in the garage, which is perfect (easy to wipe down). For a simpler process, you can just organize and sanitize everything on the front walkway.

STEP 2 Take everything out of the bags at your cleaning station. Get rid of disposable bags, and toss reusable bags in the laundry to be washed with hot water and detergent.

STEP 3 Sort your groceries, according to the category container (or lack thereof) or by the "type" of food. Try lumping it into two categories, cold stuff and shelf stable, safe stowing the cold stuff and perishables first.

STEP 4 Wipe down packaged products. You can use Lysol wipes to give your packages and products a quick wipe down. There's no need to spray them with aerosol disinfectants. Save that for your household uses (like door knobs and toilet seats). Let the products dry before handling them again. Yes, cardboard and paper packaging will be a little messed up after a sanitizing wipedown, and if you don't want that, there is an option for shelf stable products (things that don't need to go into the fridge or freezer right away). Or, you can quarantine your products. Leave your shelf-stable products in the garage a few days, and any viral organisms on their packaging will die.

STEP 5 Put it away. With clean hands, put away your disinfected products. If you have household helpers, they can take the items that have been wiped down (after the products dry). Or you can do it all. Either way, you are minimizing your risks and that's a beautiful thing these days.

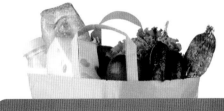

11 MAKE YOUR OWN WIPES

If you are out of Lysol wipes, make your own bleach wipe. Blend 2 teaspoons of bleach with 6 tablespoons of water, then apply this to a washcloth to wipe down your products.

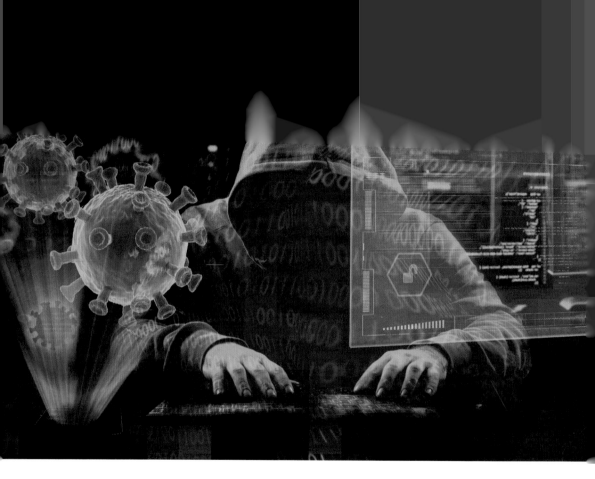

13 DON'T GET SCAMMED

Fraudsters and criminals won't pass up an opportunity to take advantage of those who are scared and vulnerable during a pandemic, so keep these things on your radar.

REJECT SNAKE OIL REMEDIES While there's a lot to be said for natural products that support healing and boost your

Unfortunately, criminals have been appearing at peoples' doors and claiming that they are from a health organization, only to barge into the house for a home invasion style of robbery. Face it, none of us are going to have the "President of the CDC" banging on our doors at 10 o'clock at night. In simple terms, don't answer the door for anyone during a

14 FACT-CHECK THE NEWS

Even before an epidemic is formally declared, you can expect to be overloaded with information from various sources such as the news media, Twitter, Facebook, and directly from your friends and neighbors. Everyone will have an opinion and suggestions for what to do, and often you'll get contradictory information—which makes everything more confusing and stressful. Here are some simple ways to make sense of all the noise.

CHECK YOUR SOURCES Be skeptical of news sources you've never heard of before. Who the heck is "True Virus Times," anyway, and why are they saying that spinach can cure you of whatever ails you? See if you can find reporting on the same information from other news sources.

KNOW THE DIFFERENCE Opinion pieces, letters to the editor, and talk shows are generally not credible sources of news.

INVESTIGATE EXTREME CLAIMS Rumor may be passed off as fact. Double check information to make sure it's not a rumor. Especially when people start feeling desperate, an irresponsible rumor can cause real harm.

CHECK THE DATE Sometimes articles that appear related from years earlier get carelessly reposted as current news. Avoid adding to the confusion by at least checking the date before you hit "share."

FACT CHECK Even trusted news sources can sometimes be wrong, especially in a fast-developing situation such as a spreading illness. Trust but verify with websites dedicated to fact checking or with respected international news sources like the Associated Press or Reuters.

CHECK YOUR BIAS Be aware of the human tendency to accept information as true simply because it seems to confirm your own beliefs.

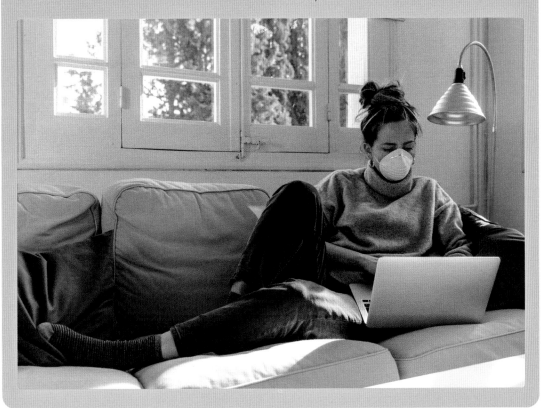

15 FACE YOUR FEAR

So many people are afraid during an emergency . . . and most people consider fear to be a bad thing, like some kind of liability or an unpleasantness that we should minimize in our lives. Our instinct of fear, however unflattering, is actually a very helpful tool when used in small doses. Sure, we're all supposed to laugh in the face of danger and never get frightened over anything, but that's just Hollywood brainwashing. We've all been scared, plenty of times in our lives, and the thing is that the right amount of fear is a good thing. And even though it's true that unbridled fear can become a hazard in a life or death crisis, fear can also save us. Here's why fear is our friend, but panic is our enemy.

ACCEPT YOUR FEARS Fear is our natural instinct concerning dangerous things. Our fear of heights keeps us from falling to our death, when it's working properly. Our fear of snakes keeps us from getting bitten, or at least it's supposed to. And similarly, our fear of COVID-19 keeps (most of us) from licking doorknobs in public places. That's right, fear keeps us safe! And when that fear is kept under control, it's working *for* us. But when we become overly stressed or fearful, we are often at the mercy of the cocktail of hormones and chemicals that pump through our bodies. It's quite common that this flush of hormones will lead to panic, which is definitely working against us.

DON'T PANIC! Panic can be described an unrestrained, illogical, and unthinking fear that is a common response to crisis. This reaction can manifest itself in many ways. If you panic, you may run around frantically. Or you may be frozen

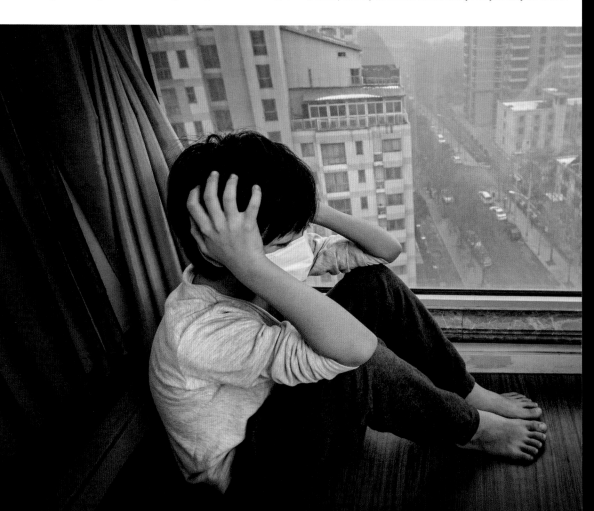

in fear and unable to move. You may even become overwhelmed by emotion. Any of these responses could get you into more trouble, and then you'll have a whole new set of problems. But if you use your fear as a tool, and hold panic at bay–then you are the master of your fear (and not the other way around).

KEEP IT TOGETHER The best way to avoid panicking in any stressful, overwhelming situation is to focus on something small that you can control, like performing a helpful task. This directs your mind away from the frightening issue and allows you to start thinking constructively again. Being wrapped up in a global pandemic is a scary thing, but if you focus on the things that you can control, your fears and worries can be held in check.

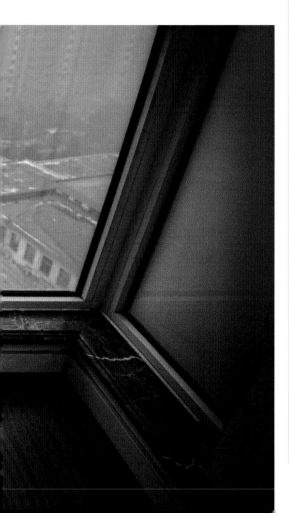

16 KEEP YOUR DISTANCE

By now, you'd have to have been hiding under a rock not to have heard of "social distancing." (Which, by the way, if you have been hiding under a rock, congratulations! You're doing a great job–now stay there!) The basic rule is to stay at least 6 feet (2 meters) away from anyone you're not already quarantined with. That sounds simple enough, but when the guy behind you in line at Target starts edging into your airspace, how close is too close? Here are some handy visuals that may not make it any easier to tell, but will possibly make it more amusing. Maybe (depending on where you live, how closely you paid attention to you history classes, and what you like to eat for lunch), it'll be easier to picture one adult gator, one Abraham Lincoln (you get almost an extra foot of safety if you include his hat!), or six delicious Subway sandwiches.

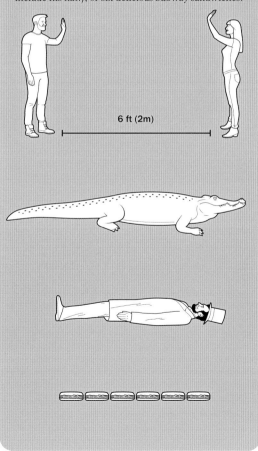

6 ft (2m)

17 WATCH THE ATTITUDE

A positive attitude in the face of adversity may be one of the most important skills to master. It is also one of the hardest, but so very worth the trouble. Think of your attitude as a lens that you are looking through. It controls your perception of any situation, and this impacts your outcome. For example, if you have a sour and negative attitude about our current pandemic situation, you'll be miserable and you'll also make everyone around you miserable. If you can look for positives in the situation, and keep an upbeat attitude, then you'll have a better day and a better outcome. The "glass" really is half-full, you just need to figure out how and believe it. Try practicing an "attitude of gratitude" in your daily routine. Reflect on the things that you are glad to have and allow that gratitude to uplift you. Your attitude controls so much of your mind and your emotions. Remember: If you don't control your attitude, it will control you.

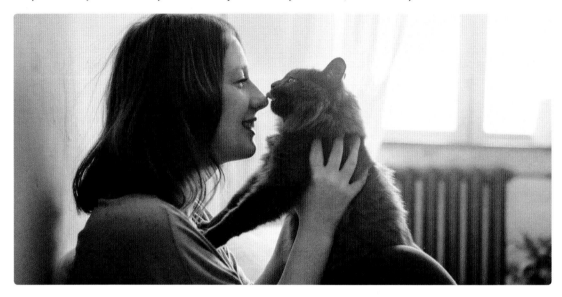

18 CULTIVATE YOUR SURVIVOR MENTALITY

Like it or not, the current pandemic is forcing us all to think about survival skills and become more self-reliant, but providing for yourself isn't always about lighting fires, building huts or making traps. Self-reliance is about enduring, through any crisis or emergency. It's not just one skill, or even a handful of skills. At its core, self-reliance is a mindset, and it's something we teach as the "survivor mentality" in books and classes. The survivor mentality is so important, in fact, that we both begin and end certain classes with the topic. So what is your survivor mentality? It's a collection of mental, emotional, psychological, and intellectual attributes that directly impact your survival. These include (but are not limited to): attitude, work ethic, adaptability, creativity, mental toughness, motivation, and tenacity. These are the things that our ancestors needed to survive and we still need these attributes to make it through tough times. We'll cover many these separate aspects of the survivor mentality in this book, but for now, focus on your attitude (since it governs so many other things)"

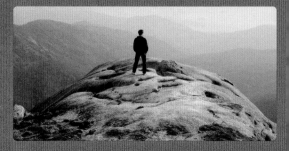

19 DON'T DESPAIR

We're in the midst of a pandemic, and anyone who is paying attention should be distressed right now. In any crisis, declining mental health is a risk that we all face. In fact, it would be rare for someone in a crisis would retain 100% of their normal mental health and emotional state. Consider the fatigue, worry, withdrawal from addictive substances, isolation, a lack of sound sleep, the changes in diet, and emotional stress in an emergency. Any regular person should be a train wreck. With this in mind, carefully monitor yourself and those around you for depression, anger, frustration, hyperactivity, feelings of intense guilt, ideas of suicide, and any irrational behavior. Do whatever you can to avoid shutting down while you're on lockdown. Reach out and get help, for yourself and those you care about.

20 LEARN FROM HISTORY

If you're been paying attention, you've been seeing warnings about the mighty power of tiny germs for years—and now, sadly, those warnings are proving true. Yes, this is a serious illness we are facing, but I'd encourage you to look for the "silver lining" in this pandemic—it could have been a much nastier bug. Covid-19 is a horrible disease, and it may take some of our loved ones away from us before this pandemic is over. This situation, however, could have easily been a bio-weapon attack (like smallpox released in every major city) or the natural spread of a more deadly disease (like Ebola or Marberg hemorrhagic fever). Here's just one example of how it could have been worse. Almost exactly a hundred years ago, the Spanish Influenza pandemic killed somewhere between 40 million and 100 million people worldwide, and infected more than 500 million people across the globe. This especially deadly form of H1N1 influenza virus began killing people in January 1918, and continued until December 1920. Yes, our current situation is scary, it won't be over soon, and most experts agree that it will get worse before it gets better—nevertheless, count your blessings. This situation could have been so much worse and we could be facing a much deadlier foe right now.

BLACK DEATH

THE NUMBERS The Black Plague (aka Black Death) hit Europe in 1347, and over the next decade killed between 100 and 200 million people—roughly half Europe's population.

CAUSE The bacteria *Yersinia pestis* is believed to be the culprit behind this unprecedented loss of life, hitching a ride to Europe on flea-infested rats.

SYMPTOMS The plague can manifest in three different ways. Bubonic plague causes swollen lymph nodes throughout the body. Septicemic plague causes bleeding from orifices. Pneumonic plague attacks the lungs and is the most dangerous plague (as it can easily be spread by coughing). All plague forms present with fever, chills, weakness, and other flu-like symptoms.

CHANCE OF RECURRENCE *Yersinia pestis* still exists in nature and still affects thousands of people worldwide, but these days it can be easily treated with antibiotics and this is unlikely to kill multitudes ever again.

"SPANISH" FLU

THE NUMBERS The influenza pandemic of 1918 (which actually began in Kansas) killed somewhere between 40 million and 100 million people worldwide, and infected more than 500 million people across the globe.

CAUSE This especially deadly form of H1N1 influenza virus began killing people in January 1918, and continued until December 1920.

SYMPTOMS This flu had all the typical symptoms (fever, nausea, diarrhea, and body aches) but it also had two unusual aspects, a high mortality rate and the fact that healthy young adults were the primary fatalities.

CHANCE OF RECURRENCE The countless strains of H1N1 influenza virus are still going strong today and there's little that modern medicine can do to fight it. An episode like the 1918 flu certainly could recur. In June 2009, a new strain of H1N1 received pandemic status as it spread worldwide, and killed 17,000 by early 2010.

SMALLPOX

THE NUMBERS Smallpox has killed untold millions of people in the last few millennium, and between 300 million and 500 million people in the 20th Century. Thanks to vaccinations, the last case in the United States happened in 1949, and the last case on earth occurred in Somalia in 1977.

CAUSE Smallpox is a disease caused by either of two viral species, *Variola major* and *Variola minor*.

SYMPTOMS The disease begins with fever and vomiting, followed by mouth sores and a unique skin rash, consisting of fluid-filled bumps that are dented in the center.

CHANCE OF RECURRENCE In 1980, the World Health Assembly declared smallpox eradicated; no cases of naturally occurring smallpox have happened since. Now for the bad news: Samples of smallpox have gone missing from storage over the years, and it's on the radar as a possible bioweapon.

21 OVERREACT (A LITTLE)

Now, to be very clear, we're not suggesting that you become a paranoid hypochondriac, hiding from the light of day. But as one of the memes that circulated as COVID-19 was starting to hit the U.S. went, "If we act quickly now, and nothing bad happens, we run the terrible danger of looking like fools. If we don't act, and it is that bad, we risk something much worse." Err on the side of caution when the stakes are high.

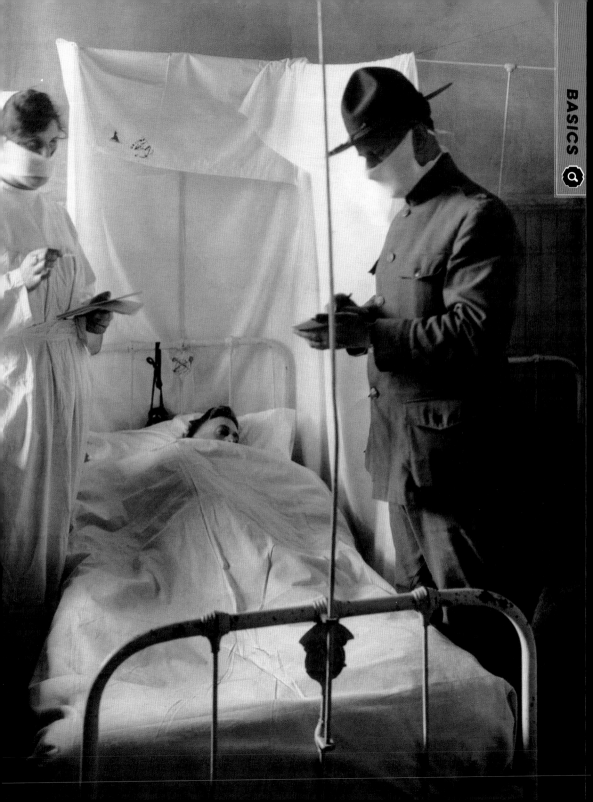

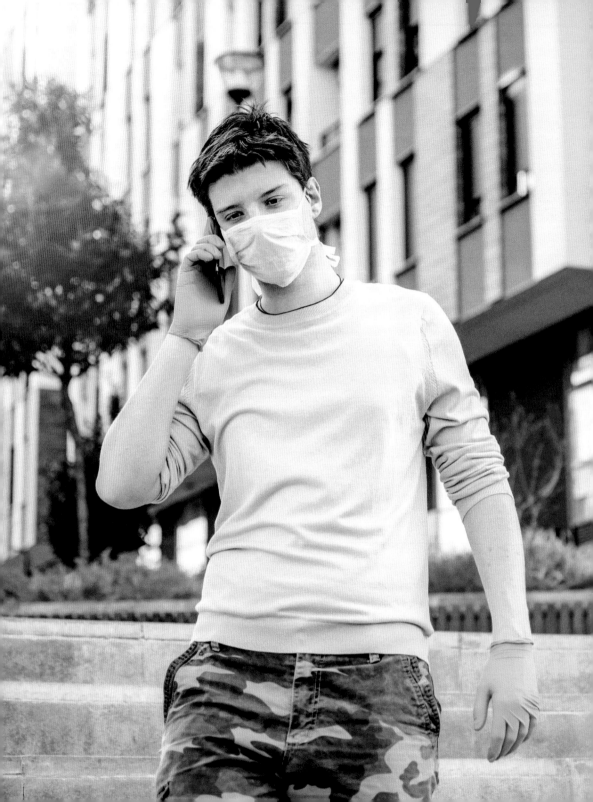

GEAR UP

Expensive gear doesn't replace good planning, but if you're smart about putting together the right equipment, that's half the battle. Indeed, if you plan carefully, you won't need—or spend—as much as you might think.

Chances are, if you're reading this book you already have some disaster gear in your kit. If so, read on for tips for some gear you may not have thought about yet. And if you're just starting to plan, then this is a great place to get serious about what you need.

FIRST AID KIT While having a well-stocked first aid or emergency response bag won't provide the kind of advanced life support needed if you get infected during a pandemic, it can keep you out of the urgent care clinic so you can lower your chances of exposure in a high-risk environment. And really, every home should have a good kit regardless.

PERSONAL PROTECTIVE EQUIPMENT Medical PPE is obviously super important in an epidemic, but since it's also very useful in almost all other disaster scenarios, adding this to your supplies is essential. When you combine medical PPE with other gear such as work gloves and helmets, you can mix and match your PPE for the task at hand.

SAFETY KNOW-HOW All the gear in the world won't save you if you don't have good pandemic hygiene, which includes washing your hands, practicing social distancing, and keeping common surfaces disinfected. PPE in a pandemic is your last line of defense, so don't think of it as your armor as much as a critical backup.

22 SUIT UP FOR SAFETY

It's counterintuitive, but personal protective equipment (PPE) is not a good source of safety—it's actually considered your last line of defense under normal circumstances. In traditional risk management, the best way to handle any risk is to eliminate it entirely, or replace it with a safer option before you have to engage with it. Administrative controls can also be used to raise awareness through the use of signs and safety monitors.

However, in a disaster situation, personal protective equipment may be your only line of defense, which is why it's so important to have access to PPE. It's also important to assign somebody to take the role of safety monitor, in order to help to maintain safety in circumstances where better options do not exist.

23 MASK UP

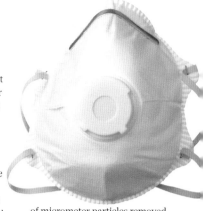

Disasters (and everyday projects) frequently involve exposure to harmful chemicals and toxins, but a mask goes far in protecting your lungs and health. Respirators and dust masks come in a variety of types and ratings. Particulate filters, including dust masks, are disposable or have replacement filters. They protect from airborne particles—including dust, mists, liquids, and some fumes—but not gases or vapors. Not all are created equal, so be sure your mask is the right one for the task.

Particulate filters are rated by the National Institute of Occupational Safety and Health (NIOSH), according to their capacity. The ratings have both a letter and number: N (not oil-proof), R (oil-resistant up to 8 hours), and P (oil-proof beyond 8 hours). Particulate filters are rated 95, 97, or 100, corresponding to the percentage of micrometer particles removed. Filters rated 100 are considered high-efficiency (HE or HEPA) filters.

The most common rating for a disposable dust mask is N95, which filters 95 percent of non-oil-based airborne particles. N95 covers basic but essential safety needs such as mold, allergens, or airborne diseases. If you need the highest level of protection in the widest variety of situations, go for P100.

24 WEAR IT PROPERLY

For the best fit and safety, there are a few useful tips to follow when wearing protective masks.

Durable half or full masks provide a better fit and protection, but disposable masks will be easier to find, however they won't seal as well. Disposable masks with an exhalation valve will make breathing easier. For higher-risk environments, choose a full face mask and disinfect after each use. Masks with an exhalation valve may make breathing easier. For higher-risk environments (such as asbestos), choose a non-disposable mask with sealing gaskets.

25 PUT THE RIGHT ONE ON

This chart will help you decide what kind of mask you should wear, depending on the substance in question.

RATING	SUBSTANCES
N95 OR HIGHER	Allergens, bacteria and viruses, bleach, dust, non-asbestos fibers, insulation, mold, pollen, debris from sanding and welding
N100 OR HEPA	Asbestos, lead
R95 OR HIGHER	Paint, pesticides, sprays

26 DON A MASK

Wearing an N95 mask can be a vital step in keeping yourself and others healthy. (That said, if you're not a medical professional, and live in one of the many areas where supplies are desperately short, do seriously consider donating your stash to a local hospital). If you can isolate in your home, the donation could literally save a precious life. If you are an essential worker, or immune suppressed, or if your area is not experiencing shortages, a properly fitted N95 is definitely your best option. Here's how to don it properly, for optimal safety, and how to remove it as well.

Here's how to don it properly, for optimal safety, and how to remove it as well.

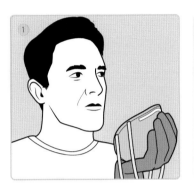

STEP 1 Always wash your hands thoroughly first, then hold the mask in the palm of your hand with the straps over your fingers and the mask's exterior facing the floor.

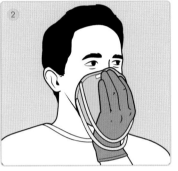

STEP 2 Place the mask onto your face, holding it so that it's fully covering your nose and mouth.

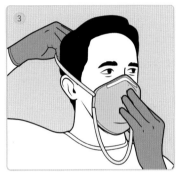

STEP 3 Pull the top strap up and over top of your head, and secure it behind your head, resting as snugly as possible above your ears.

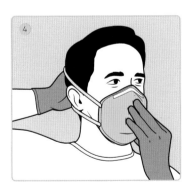

STEP 4 Take the lower strap and pull it over to place it behind your head and below your ears.

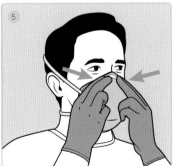

STEP 5 Mold the chevron-shaped metal nose piece of the respirator over the bridge of your nose to obtain a tight fit.

Finally, place your hands gently on the N95 mask and exhale. Adjust straps if the mask shifts during exhalation or if air escapes from the edges of the mask.

PRO TIPS

- Never touch the inside of mask, so as to avoid contaminating it.

- When removing a mask, always be sure to remove your gloves first so as to avoid contaminating it (after all, you're wearing your gloves to protect you, so just assume that they're contaminated by the time you need to remove the mask).

27 SEW A MASK

There are a lot of DIY mask patters out there. Here's one you can make with just a bit of sewing savvy.

STEP 1 Wash and iron your fabric, then fold it in half so you have double layers 6.5 x 9.5 inches. Then cut along the fold to make two equal rectangles.

STEP 2 Cut 4 thin pieces of material, about 18 inches long and 3/4 inches wide. Fold each piece of fabric twice lengthwise, then one more to tuck the rough edges inside. Sew a straight line along the middle. This will prevent the ties from having frayed edges. You can also use elastic, or even shoelaces.

STEP 3 Take one of your rectangle fabric layers. With the right side facing you, pin down the fabric ties, one piece per corner. Wrap each tie around itself to keep it away from the edges.

STEP 4 Take the second layer of fabric and line it up with the first. The "right sides" (or patterned side) of the fabric ties or elastics. Secure the fabric sandwich together with pins.

STEP 5 From the rough midpoint, sew a straight line across the mask, about 14 inches from above the bottom edge of the fabric, toward the bottom left-hand corner. Make sure that the elastic or fabric ties are secured in the corners, sandwiched by your two layers of fabric, as you sew over the ends. You want to make sure your needle goes through the three pieces: the top layer, the end of the fabric tie, and the bottom layer. Add a couple stitches forward and backward (in both directions) to secure your ties in place.

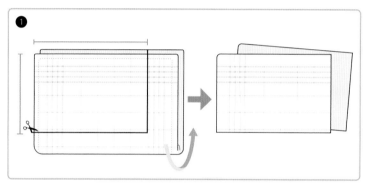

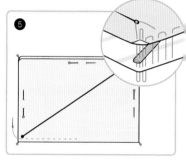

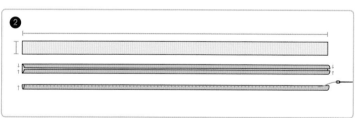

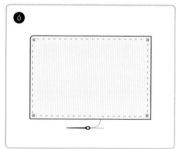

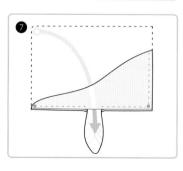

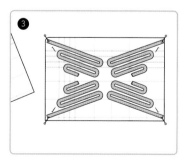

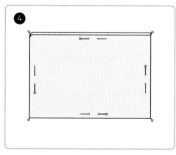

STEP 6 Sew almost all the way around the rectangle., leaving a half-inch gap that you'll use to pull the mask right-side out.

STEP 7 Carefully turn the mask right-side out by pulling it through the gap you left in your stitching.

STEP 8 Pull your ties out of the way, and smooth or kiron the mask flat.

STEP 9 Fold a series of three or four horizontal pleats and pin them down.

(This step is optional, but it really helps the mask conform to the wearer's face.)

STEP 10 Stitch around your mask's edges one last time, to anchor the pleats and close your gaps. Voila! Now you can walk the streets feeling both safer and more stylish, espeically if you sew a mask for every mood!

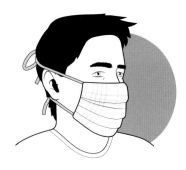

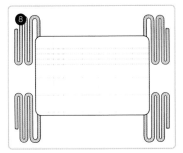

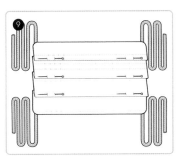

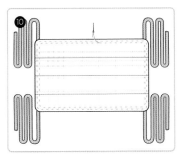

28 BRIEF YOURSELF

Maybe you can't sew. Maybe you need a mask pronto. Maybe you've just always wanted an excuse to wear your undies on your head. We don't judge (so long as they're clean, of course.) Here's a wrap-and-go mask that's, well, better than nothing.

Start by placing one leg of a pair of stretchy boxer briefs over you lower face. Now, reach back, grab the elastic waistband, and pull it up over your forehead, tucking the back leg neatly inside your new burnoose. Tighten around your face and wear with pride.

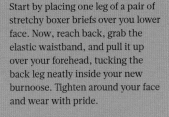

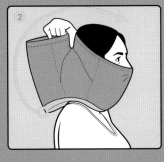

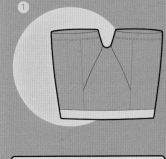

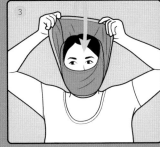

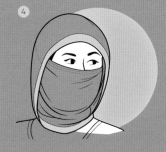

29 MAKE A CHEAP SUIT

Concerned about the flu or some even more sinister pathogens? You'll need the right supplies for protection. You can use some or all of these simple items to create a DIY protective suit, should the horseman of pestilence ride through your town.

STEP 1 Start by hitting your local hardware store for a set of Tyvek coveralls. These are tough, tear-proof, and almost waterproof. They're commonly available and can also be purchased with head and shoe covers.

STEP 2 Grab a little duct tape to tape the joints of your suit.

STEP 3 Add a standard medical mask, such as an N95 mask or even an N99. Grab a big box of them at one of those warehouse stores, and you'll have plenty extra for other people to wear.

STEP 4 Add work goggles to the outfit, especially ones with an anti-fog coating and vents.

STEP 5 Finally, nitrile gloves will protect your hands, without causing latex allergies.

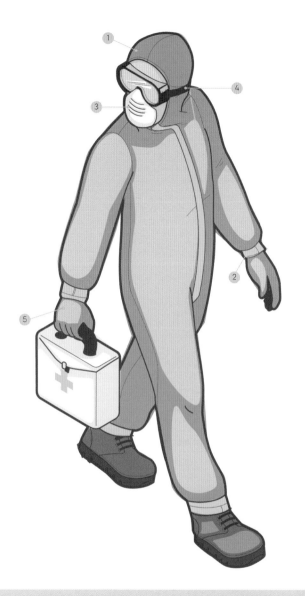

30 LAYER YOUR PROTECTION

Disposable filter masks are one of the cheapest defenses against airborne pathogens. The common N95 mask protects against 95% of the particulates larger than 0.3 microns in size. The next masks are N99 masks (99% effective) and N100 masks (99.7% effective). But none of these help much if they don't make a tight seal around your nose and mouth because of facial hair.

Whether it's just shaving stubble or a full beard, air will seek the path of least resistance—gaps created between your mask and your skin. But here's a helpful way to better protect your mask. Put on a cloth mask over your N95 mask to protect you, and your mask, a bit more. And every little bit will help.

Wondering about R and P rated masks? They are rated for industrial use, but they will also protect you just as well from diseases as the N rated masks will do.

31 GET GOOD GLOVES

There is a dizzying array of glove options to keep you safe in the field, and each type of glove protects against different hazards. Get to know the pros and cons of a few basic glove types that you're likely to consider for your PPE needs.

For medical gloves [A] your best material choice is nitrile. These gloves are safe for people with latex allergies—an increasing concern in health care. For improved dexterity, stock up on textured gloves. You can also put on vinyl or polyethylene (plastic) gloves, but they are less protective. Avoid using high-priced durable gloves because, once they have been contaminated with bodily fluids, the gloves are no longer considered safe and should be discarded.

For a general-purpose work glove [B], consider a modern hybrid type that may combine synthetic fibers with leather, plastic, and other materials for the best comfort, dexterity, durability, and grip. The trade-off for this balance is that these hybrids are outdone by gloves specifically designed for just one or two factors. For example, a pair of heavy canvas or leather gloves will be more durable than hybrid work gloves. However, heavy materials need to be broken in, can be incredibly uncomfortable to wear, and may cause blisters or abrasions on your hands.

Tactical gloves [C], sometimes also referred to as police gloves, are good general-purpose wear when not giving first aid or doing search-and-rescue work. They offer a variety of protection such as Kevlar linings to make them puncture- or cut-resistant while also providing excellent grip, warmth and dexterity. Avoid riot gloves or search gloves, since the former are aggressive and can suggest to others that you're looking for a fight, while the latter offer you very little in the way of protection or warmth, since their primary function is sensitive dexterity while frisking subjects.

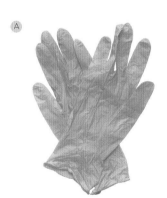
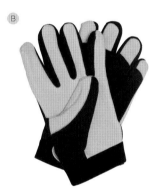
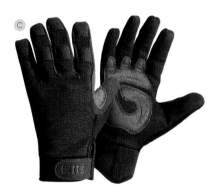

32 CHANGE GLOVES OFTEN

Any of the disposable medical gloves degrade over time, which reduces their effectiveness in protecting you from potentially contagious body fluids while rendering first aid. While standard procedure is to change gloves after every patient in medical contexts, in other situations people tend to wear the same pair of gloves for many hours at a time, but this is not recommended. Oils from your hands, skin lotion, chemicals, disinfectants, heat, and other elements all degrade the protection of your disposable gloves. When in doubt, replace your gloves!

33 DON'T BE A HERO

Equipping yourself with all of the very best of the personal protective equipment may make you feel like a superhero, but, the reality is, none of this is armor. You should still approach hazards as if you have no PPE on. This way, you're consciously avoiding any overconfidence you might gain from all the gear that you are wearing. And overconfidence can kill you as it's killed others in the past. Remember that PPE is your last resort for safety, and the best way to handle risk is to avoid it entirely whenever possible.

These days, we mainly think of PPE in terms of avoiding contagion—for obvious reasons! However, it can be helpful to understand the larger world of protective gear, because you never know what the future may bring.

PREPARED

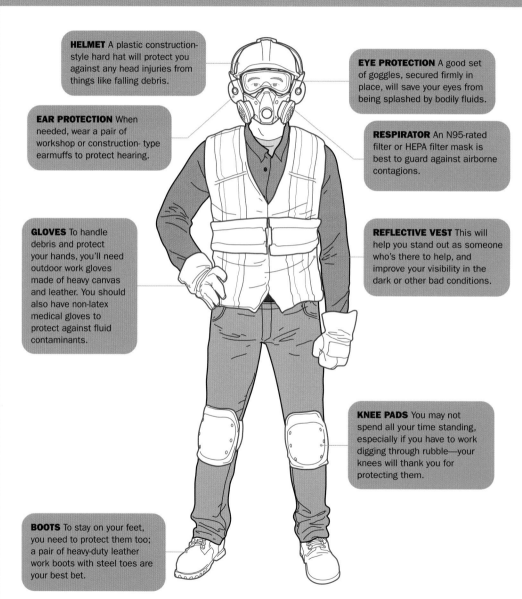

HELMET A plastic construction-style hard hat will protect you against any head injuries from things like falling debris.

EAR PROTECTION When needed, wear a pair of workshop or construction- type earmuffs to protect hearing.

GLOVES To handle debris and protect your hands, you'll need outdoor work gloves made of heavy canvas and leather. You should also have non-latex medical gloves to protect against fluid contaminants.

EYE PROTECTION A good set of goggles, secured firmly in place, will save your eyes from being splashed by bodily fluids.

RESPIRATOR An N95-rated filter or HEPA filter mask is best to guard against airborne contagions.

REFLECTIVE VEST This will help you stand out as someone who's there to help, and improve your visibility in the dark or other bad conditions.

KNEE PADS You may not spend all your time standing, especially if you have to work digging through rubble—your knees will thank you for protecting them.

BOOTS To stay on your feet, you need to protect them too; a pair of heavy-duty leather work boots with steel toes are your best bet.

IMPROVISED

EYE PROTECTION Goggles are ideal, but if nothing else, a pair of sunglasses or regular glasses will help protect your eyes.

RESPIRATOR A painter's dust mask or bandanna is not the most protective, especially against infectious substances, but it'll do in a pinch.

VEST If you don't have a reflective vest, look for something else bright that stands out well, like a neon-colored or tie-dyed shirt.

BOOTS Rain boots or hiking boots are not as sturdy as work boots or similar footwear; nonetheless, they'll cover your feet better than flip-flops or sneakers.

HELMET Any head protection is better than nothing if you're in a dangerous zone during some kind of unrest. Even a bike helmet can be useful.

EAR PROTECTION Disposable foam earplugs will protect your hearing, though keeping them clean and trying not to lose them when you remove them briefly is a hassle.

GLOVES A set of gardening gloves and/or a pair of rubber kitchen or cleaning gloves will help to keep your hands safe.

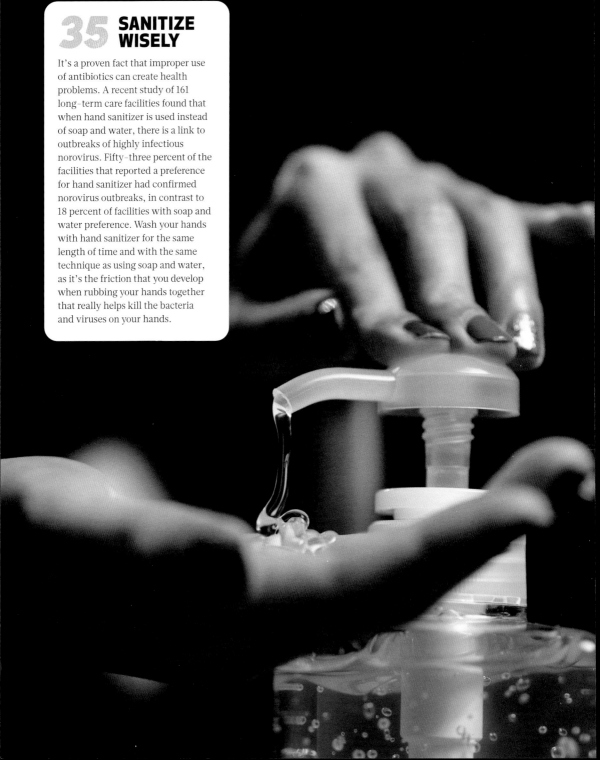

35 SANITIZE WISELY

It's a proven fact that improper use of antibiotics can create health problems. A recent study of 161 long-term care facilities found that when hand sanitizer is used instead of soap and water, there is a link to outbreaks of highly infectious norovirus. Fifty-three percent of the facilities that reported a preference for hand sanitizer had confirmed norovirus outbreaks, in contrast to 18 percent of facilities with soap and water preference. Wash your hands with hand sanitizer for the same length of time and with the same technique as using soap and water, as it's the friction that you develop when rubbing your hands together that really helps kill the bacteria and viruses on your hands.

36 MAKE DIY HAND SANITIZER

We're all familiar with that gooey disinfectant gel which is your best line of defense when you can't wash your hands with soap and water.

But what if your local stores have all run out of the goopy good stuff? Luckily it's easy to make, provided you have just a few simple ingredients. The primary component is rubbing alcohol, also known as isopropyl. CDC guidelines suggest sterilizing with at least 60% alcohol solutions; higher is always better, so get 99% if you can. Ethanol (a.k.a. grain alcohol) can also work in a pinch, but just like isopropyl, it must be at least 120 Proof (60% ABV) or higher.

THE FAST-AND-DIRTY RECIPE You can make a simple hand sanitizer with just two ingredients: alcohol and aloe vera gel. Combine the two in a 2:1 ratio, mix thoroughly, let sit for 72 hours, then use! The aloe vera will even help keep your hands moisturized since alcohol is astringent, but can leave your hands a bit sticky afterward.

THE TRIED-AND-TRUE METHOD For a version of your own homemade hand sanitizer that's less tacky-feeling after use (and more effective to boot), combine rubbing alcohol, glycerin, and 3% hydrogen peroxide solution in a 12:1:2 ratio. If the alcohol percentage is lower than 99%, ensure that the final mix is still 60% alcohol or higher—this formula has a 75% ratio of alcohol to other ingredients, while 91% isopropyl would net a 73% solution. This version is thinner than the aloe vera version, and works best in an automatic spray dispenser or handheld spray bottle; from there it can be sprayed directly onto surfaces or hands, or onto paper towels.

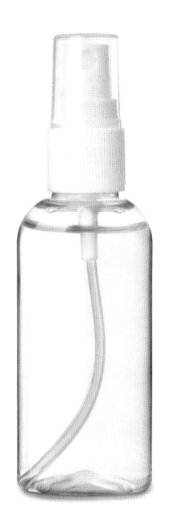

37 AVOID TOXIC COMBINATIONS

We know it's tempting to take a look at the many household cleansers and sanitizing products in your cabinet and wonder if you could combine a super-sanitizing solution. The short answer: You might, but the mix would also probably kill you along with the pathogens. Alcohol and peroxide work together just fine under most conditions (which is why they can be combined in the formula in the previous article). Everything else? Not so much.

Bleach and ammonia combined produce chloramine, a toxic gas that causes chest pain, shortness of breath, and fluid buildup in the lungs. Vinegar or other acidic products mixed with bleach will create chlorine gas, which can be deadly when inhaled and can also form hydrochloric acid vapor. Bleach and rubbing alcohol together create chloroform, a carcinogen (which itself oxidizes, eventually turning into hydrochloric acid vapor and phosgene, another toxic substance). Even a simple combination of vinegar and peroxide creates peroxyacetic acid, a severe irritant to the eyes and respiratory system.

These are just some of the most common combinations, but the idea is simple: Don't mix cleansers and sanitizers. Ultimately any pathogens you face can be most easily defeated by the simplest measures—sanitation, isolation, and hand washing.

38 BUILD YOUR FIRST AID KIT

If you're the type of person who's always asking for a bandage or aspirin, it's time to get it together. Create a kit that includes the following items.

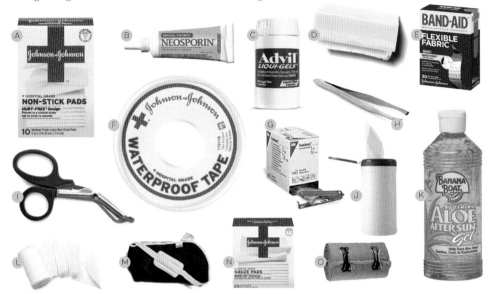

A. Non-stick dressings	F. Medical tape	J. Disinfectant towelettes
B. Antibacterial ointment	G. Splint materials (inflatable or rigid wood/plastic)	K. Aloe vera gel
C. Anti-inflammatory drugs		L. Gauze roller bandages
D. Surgical scrub brush	H. Tweezers	M. Arm sling
E. Adhesive bandages, including butterfly strips	I. Medical shears (a.k.a. EMT scissors)	N. Sterile compress
		O. Elastic roller bandages

If you've got the know-how (perhaps with EMS or some other medical training) you might add these to your medical supplies. Some "jump bags" are even prepacked with these items—and many more.

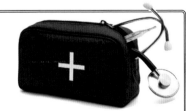

- Trauma pads (some even help speed blood clotting)
- CPR mask
- Chemical hot and cold packs
- Normal saline (for rinsing injuries)
- EpiPens (for anaphylactic allergic reactions)

- Stethoscope
- Nitrile gloves
- Oral glucose tubes (for diabetic emergencies)
- Activated charcoal (for ingested poisons)
- Emergency tourniquet

- Wilderness/travel medicine guidebook
- Penlight
- Blood pressure cuff

39 IMPROVISE MEDICAL SUPPLIES

In an emergency, having the medical gear you need can be a godsend. But what if you're forced to make do with the materials at hand? There are plenty of DIY options.

BUTTERFLY STRIPS Small pieces of tape can be snipped with scissors to create butterfly dressings to hold cuts closed. Snip them twice on each of the long sides, and fold the middle under to create a non-stick section that would float over the laceration.

DRESSINGS Although they are not sterile, feminine hygiene pads can provide you with a decent wound dressing. Tampons are a bit more sterile, and they can be laid sideways on a wound. Strap down any of these dressings with clean cloth strips, tape, or any other binding you have at hand.

INSECT STING RELIEF Meat tenderizer is made of enzymes that break down tough steak proteins—and those found in bug venom! Mix the tenderizer and a drop or two of water into a paste and apply it directly to the sting or bite. It won't help a rattlesnake bite, but this mixture can somewhat relieve the pain from hornet, wasp, scorpion, and ant stings.

SPLINTS Splints are one of the easier bits of medical gear to improvise. Your goal is immobilization, which can be achieved with any number of rigid items and binding materials, such as a board and some duct tape. Make sure you stuff adequate padding inside the splint to properly stabilize the limb and ease your patient's pain—use crumpled toilet paper or newspaper, spare clothing, or anything else that works.

BURN GEL Crush an aloe vera leaf and smear the clear goop on the dressing for a burn wound and then apply. It's simple and surprisingly effective, too.

DISINFECTANT Keep infections at bay by putting straight liquor onto topical wounds, if you must. Yes, it will hurt (and can slow healing since it kills exposed tissue cells), but it's better to hurt now and heal than to let a wound become infected, which will result in a lot more pain later.

40 LEVEL UP

Remember, the first step in taking care of injuries is knowing what supplies to use and how to use them properly. This is the baseline level of what any well-prepared person should know. To take your knowledge to the next level, there are no shortage of first-responder and first-aid courses and books available. You can also inquire with your local Red Cross for information on classes.

First-aid and first-responder courses are just the beginning when learning about emergency medical treatment. Your local college or other educational institution may offer EMS classes lasting from a few weeks of accelerated training to a few months of intermittent sessions that you can fit into your schedule. These classes will not only give you training but also prepare you to acquire an EMT license.

41 CHECK VITAL SIGNS

The two most important aspects of a person's vitals are their respiration and circulation—breathing and heartbeat. To count someone's breaths, either watch for the rise and fall of his chest or listen to his breathing (with or without a stethoscope) for 15 seconds, then multiply by four (normal is 12–20 breaths per minute).

The easiest places to take someone's pulse are the wrist and the throat. For the wrist, press two fingers against the inside of the forearm, on the thumb side. Count the number of beats in 15 seconds, and multiply that by four (60 to 100 is normal). For the throat, find the Adam's apple, then move your fingers to the side just under the jaw. Press gently with two fingers, and measure the beats using the same method.

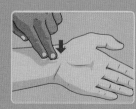
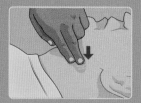

42 CREATE A CLEAN ROOM

In the event of a major epidemic, you may not have access to a modern medical facility, but you'll still need a way to quarantine sick people. Setting up an army tent in the back yard would be the safest way to separate the ill people from the healthy ones, but it's not an affordable or applicable option for most households. By contrast, an isolation room can be set up almost anywhere, cheaply and quickly. With some caution and few supplies, you can set up a "sick room" in your home to care for ill family and friends, while reducing the chance of spreading the disease throughout your group. In the early days of the COVID-19 pandemic, many folks weren't able to make it to a hospital even for family members who were not feeling well and probably contagious. Of course the best option is to have those patients under proper medical care but, if it comes down to it, here's how to set up your quarantine room.

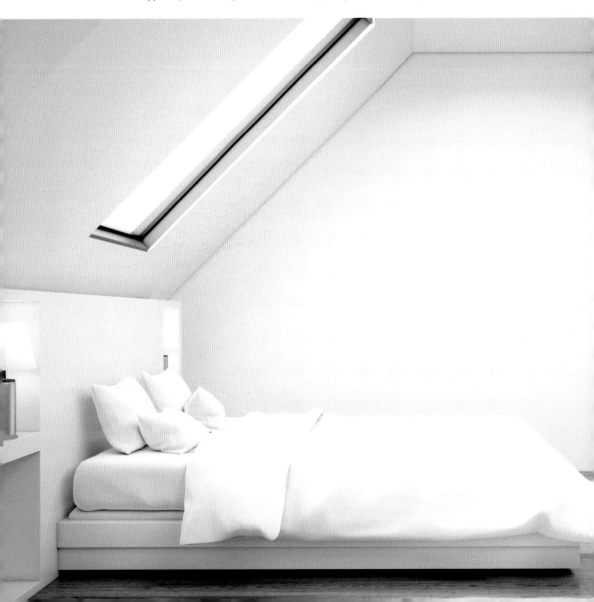

CHOOSE A SPACE Ideally, you'll have a guest room with its own bathroom, windows for ventilation, away from the main traffic areas of the home. Realistically, since most of us don't have that kind of space, you may have to settle for an out-of-the-way bedroom with a bucket for a toilet.

CONTROL AIRFLOW If your home has central air conditioning and/or heating, you'll need to block off the air flow to the isolation room. Cover floor and wall vents tightly with plastic sheets and duct tape. Never choose a room for an isolation room if it has an air return for the AC or heating system. This could suck in bacteria and viruses, and spread them throughout the home.

SUIT UP Once this room is set up, only one person should be caregiver to the infected person (or persons). They should wear coveralls, a mask, gloves, and goggles. They should have a pair of slip-on shoes, that are only to be worn in the isolation room, and that remain outside the door when not in use. An apron or smock can be made from a large trash bag by cutting arm and head holes in one end. This could go over the coveralls as extra protection from bodily fluids, or to protect your clothing if you don't have coveralls. Have your patient wear a standard surgical mask to minimize the dangerous droplets they expel from coughing and sneezing.

DISINFECT When exiting the room, spray down your protective gear with disinfectant and wait one minute before disrobing from contaminated protective gear. Outside of the isolation room door, place a trash can with a lid. This will be the receptacle for anything contaminated by contact with the infected person or the room. Disinfecting spray should also be stationed outside the door. It should be used on the trash can, the door knob, and any potentially contaminated surfaces in the isolation room and outside of it.

MAINTAIN ISOLATION Nothing inside the room should come out, if at all possible. Dishes, cups and utensils for the infected should be disposable, and discarded in a trash bag inside the isolation room. Sheets and bedding should be washed in hot water with bleach, and hung to dry in the room if possible. A sheet of plastic between the mattress and bedding will keep the mattress from absorbing blood, vomit and other bodily fluids. The isolation room should be cleaned daily, with all solid surfaces wiped down by a disinfectant.

MAKE SOME NOISE Finally, your patient should have an easy way to signal for help, as they may be too weak to call out. A bell, rattle, or some similar noise making gizmo should be with your patient's reach.

43 BUILD A BUCKET TOILET

If your quarantine room doesn't have it's own bathroom, you're going to need to create some kind of alternative toilet so that your family member can stay in the room constantly and reduce the risk of infection to your healthy loved ones. This can be done with a simple short-term solution—the bucket toilet.

Supplies:
- **Thick plastic trash bags**
- **A small bag of kitty litter**
- **Toilet paper**
- **Duct tape**
- **A permanent marker**
- **Disposable gloves**
- **Hand sanitizer**
- **A 5-gallon (20-liter) painter's bucket**

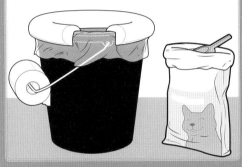

This "indoor outhouse" isn't fancy, but it's very useful – for pandemics and many other disaster settings. The listed items can be sealed inside the bucket to keep moisture out during storage. As an extra-comfort option, you can buy a special toilet seat from disaster supply stores that's designed to fit on the bucket or you can use foam pipe insulation for a soft rim.

To set up your toilet, use two trash bags to "double-bag" the inside of the bucket and secure them with duct tape. Add your seat or use the pipe insulation for a softer rim. Sprinkle some kitty litter inside (and after each use). You can even hang your TP roll on the bucket handle! Replace the bucket lid after each use. When the bucket is about half full, seal the inner bag with a knot, then tie the outer bag with another knot, then finally seal the knot with duct tape and write "Human Waste" on the duct tape with the marker. Place waste bags someplace out of the way, preferably out of direct sunlight. Check local regulations on how to properly dispose of waste, if waste management is running.

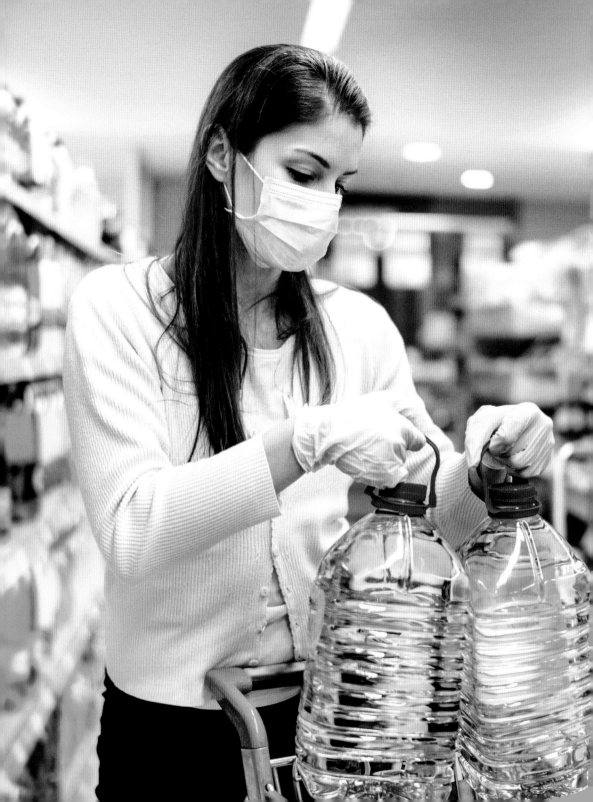

STOCK UP

For those who have never understood the merits of planning ahead or building an emergency reserve, we hope you're listening now. When you stock up on shelf-stable foods, it's like buying an edible insurance policy.

While shoppers went into panic mode in March of 2020, stripping all of the Lysol and toilet paper from grocery store shelves, the die-hard preppers were laughing all the way to the bathroom. They've known forever that you need to stockpile more than food.

MAKE SMART PURCHASES Yes, you found a case of picked pigs' feet at the almost-empty grocery store, but is that really a "win"? Even before the first hints emerge that a pandemic (or any other crisis) is headed your way, it's critical to shop wisely and avoid panic buying.

CREATE A WATER PLAN We need water every day to drink, to cook, and to perform basic hygiene. A practical person should have water stored that is ready to use, and have back-up plans for procuring more water. And to those who ask, "but why would water run short in a pandemic?" the answer is, it might not. But if anything goes wrong with the local or national infrastructure, repairs may not happen quickly. And it's not like your water stash is going to go bad if you don't use it quickly.

IMPROVISE AND OVERCOME Challenging times can inspire us to rise to meet the challenge. When you're unable to get the supplies and resources you require, an adaptive survivor can find a way to turn the stuff you have into what you need.

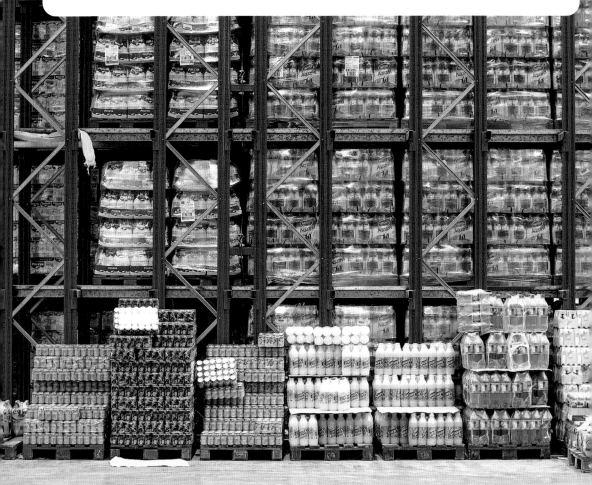

44 SHOP SMART

Get ten different disaster experts together and you'll hear at least ten different ideas to fill the perfect survival pantry. Factors include what emergency you're preparing for (pandemic? economic crash? the end times?), how many folks you need to feed, and what you like. Your postapocalyptic pantry shouldn't be all beer and cheese puffs (although the latter are great fire starters), nor do you want to spend weeks, months, or years gnawing on hardtack and tofu jerky. A good pantry plan balances out storability, nutrition, and taste. The following pages have a few guidelines to get you started.

You'll probably want to make your first trip to one of the big warehouse stores, since they tend to stock large bulk packages and have great prices. However, selection can be spotty. So, in order to fill in the gaps, look online and in specialty stores for additional items to round out your supplies.

A lot of people get superexcited about prepping and feel like they need to stock up on everything immediately. It makes more sense to build your stash a bit at a time, being sure to get what you really want and need, rather than what's on sale this week at the MegaloMart.

45 START WITH THE BASICS

It's debatable what's absolutely essential for your survival pantry, and what's a "nice to have," or even a "you stocked up on what?" Here are some pretty inarguable staples everyone should at least consider.

SALT It makes your food taste better, helps you preserve meats, and lasts pretty much forever. Natural salt and iodized salt are both great to stock. You need that iodine for thyroid health, but you'll need salt without iodine for fermenting veggies (like sauerkraut).

BAKING POWDER This pantry essential is used in cooking, but it's also good for cleaning, deodorizing, or other household chores.

FATS AND OILS Tubs of solid vegetable shortening have fairly long shelf lives. Olive oil is healthy and versatile but tends to go bad more quickly, so buy it in smaller bottles and open as needed. Coconut oil is a surprising favorite.

SUGAR AND OTHER SWEETS White sugar can be stored for a very long period if packaged right. Honey and molasses are also good to have on hand for cooking and for livening up oatmeal and the like.

RICE Like beans, rice is one of those go-to staples that has kept large portions of this planet's population alive through good times and bad. Combine with beans to boost nutrients.

BEANS Sure, beans and rice are practically a prepper cliché, but most clichés exist for a reason. Dried, beans can last for up to 30 years, they're full of nutrients, and when cooked right, they're really pretty tasty.

VITAMINS No matter how well your pantry is stocked, you may not get the variety that would be ideal in your diet. Supplement with a good multipurpose vitamin and mineral pill just to be sure.

CANNED GOODS Stock up on a good selection of fruits and vegetables—choose whatever you and your family like best, but be sure to get a variety for extra nutrition and to prevent boredom if you're eating out of your stockpiles for a while.

COFFEE AND/OR TEA Some people might class these beverages under luxuries, not essentials, but those people have never seen an addict at 6 a.m. without caffeine. Even if you're not a giant fan of coffee, it can be a fantastic trade good, so you should stock at least a few cans just in case.

DRIED FRUIT A great way to store fruit for the long-term, and a fantastic source of concentrated nutrition. A handful of raisins can sweeten your morning cereal, and some dried apricots make a nice portable source of energy. Buy them in bulk or make your own (see item 178 for instructions).

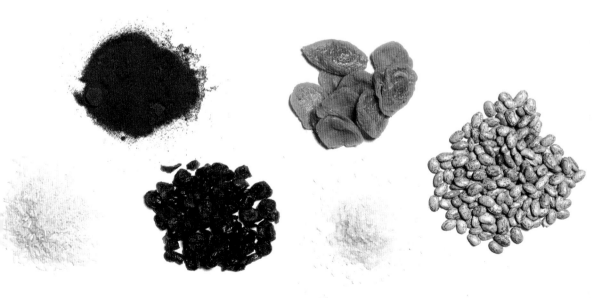

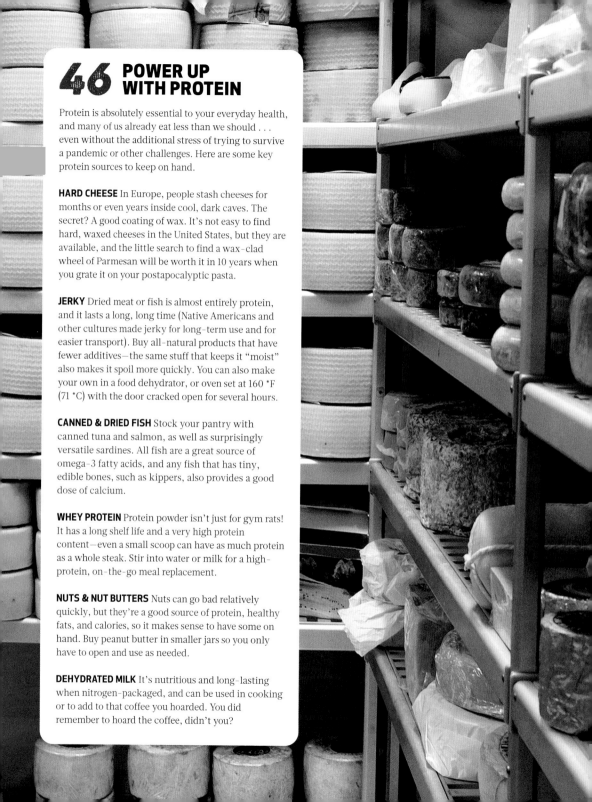

46 POWER UP WITH PROTEIN

Protein is absolutely essential to your everyday health, and many of us already eat less than we should . . . even without the additional stress of trying to survive a pandemic or other challenges. Here are some key protein sources to keep on hand.

HARD CHEESE In Europe, people stash cheeses for months or even years inside cool, dark caves. The secret? A good coating of wax. It's not easy to find hard, waxed cheeses in the United States, but they are available, and the little search to find a wax-clad wheel of Parmesan will be worth it in 10 years when you grate it on your postapocalyptic pasta.

JERKY Dried meat or fish is almost entirely protein, and it lasts a long, long time (Native Americans and other cultures made jerky for long-term use and for easier transport). Buy all-natural products that have fewer additives—the same stuff that keeps it "moist" also makes it spoil more quickly. You can also make your own in a food dehydrator, or oven set at 160 °F (71 °C) with the door cracked open for several hours.

CANNED & DRIED FISH Stock your pantry with canned tuna and salmon, as well as surprisingly versatile sardines. All fish are a great source of omega-3 fatty acids, and any fish that has tiny, edible bones, such as kippers, also provides a good dose of calcium.

WHEY PROTEIN Protein powder isn't just for gym rats! It has a long shelf life and a very high protein content—even a small scoop can have as much protein as a whole steak. Stir into water or milk for a high-protein, on-the-go meal replacement.

NUTS & NUT BUTTERS Nuts can go bad relatively quickly, but they're a good source of protein, healthy fats, and calories, so it makes sense to have some on hand. Buy peanut butter in smaller jars so you only have to open and use as needed.

DEHYDRATED MILK It's nutritious and long-lasting when nitrogen-packaged, and can be used in cooking or to add to that coffee you hoarded. You did remember to hoard the coffee, didn't you?

47 GO CARB CRAZY

The modern fear of carbs is just that . . . modern. For most of history, humans have relied on starchy foods for energy, comfort, and nutrients. And the All Grapefruit Supermodel Diet has no place in a disaster situation.

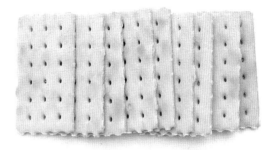

WHOLE-WHEAT FLOUR Whole-grain flour does spoil more quickly than the white stuff, but it also has a lot more nutrients. Store it carefully.

DRIED CORN This Native American staple has a very long shelf life and can be ground up to make grits, polenta, and cornbread. Or if you want to get really old-school, look into making masa harina (or just buy some premade for your pantry). This corn flour processed with lime is used to make nutritious corn tortillas.

OATMEAL Buy the whole, steel-cut oats and you have a versatile staple that can be cooked up for breakfast or used in baking to add nutrients and fiber.

CRACKERS You don't get a lot of nutrition from crackers, but they have a long shelf life, are easy to eat, and can be a good snack for kids (or grown-ups!) who need some sense of normalcy in a tough situation. Never underestimate the calming power of peanut butter and saltines!

PASTA & NOODLES Dried pasta lasts virtually forever and, if you buy the fortified kind, can be a source of some vitamins as well. Ramen noodles aren't terribly good for you, but they're easy to cook and can be a nice comfort food.

48 STASH SOME LITTLE LUXURIES

You need to eat to stay healthy, but palate fatigue will set in quick if you're living solely on whey powder and canned tomatoes. If you're going to be eating from your pantry for more than a few days, you really want to be sure it will provide variety and enjoyment as well as sheer nutrition. Even Soylent Green tastes better with a little horseradish.

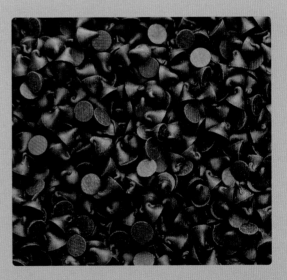

HERBS & SPICES A dash of hot sauce or a sprinkling of oregano can make a bland survival dish into a real meal. Grow fresh herbs and chile peppers in your kitchen garden, and stock your pantry with some versatile basics. Tabasco and soy sauces last virtually forever, cinnamon and ginger spice up desserts and tea, and prefab spice blends ("Italian seasoning," "Chinese five-spice powder," and the like) make flavorful cooking easy.

CONDIMENTS Most condiments spoil pretty quickly, so buy them in smaller-size bottles, and open as needed. Flavored vinegars have a very long shelf life and can liven up all kinds of dishes.

SWEETS Bags of chocolate chips and bars of high-quality chocolate last well if stored in a cool place. Chocolate syrup and cocoa powder are also good treats in tough times.

PERSONAL FAVORITES While making your bulk purchases of those essential canned tomatoes, corn, beans, and peaches, throw in some quirky indulgences that will brighten your day even if it's day 45 of shelter in place and you're going a little bonkers. That might be fancy stuffed olives in a jar, hearts of palm, pumpkin pie filling, or whatever else might lift your spirits after a week or two of oatmeal and bean soup.

49 TAKE A RATIONAL APPROACH TO RATIONING

Rationing sounds unpleasant, and it generally is. We don't have to "ration" our food, water, or other vital supplies when times are good. When things get harder, however, rationing is a very useful practice. Technically, a ration is defined as "a fixed allowance of provisions or food, especially for soldiers or sailors or for civilians during a shortage" but there's a more positive way to look at this subject. When rationing is self-imposed, it can be better defined as the collaboration between planning and self-control. Rationing is less painful, when you acquired a generous amount of supplies before the emergency. On the flip side, rationing is more painful when you have less to divide or a longer period to cover. Let's get down to the mechanics of it.

PLAN WELL The planning aspect of rationing is fairly easy and there are two ways to do it. The first option is to decide how long you want to spread out your resource and determine how much you have. Divide your resource into servings, and stick to your serving size for use. The second way to plan your rationing is to determine how much you use (by yourself or for your group) and how much you have. Calculate the servings available and see how many days it will last. Plan when those days will be (consecutive or non-consecutive), and then stick to your plan.

COUNT CALORIES Like always, just ignore the ridiculously small serving suggestions on packages, and count the calories that you need instead. Unless the third grade was the hardest four years of your life, the math should be easy.

STAY TOUGH The hard part comes when you have to exercise self-control. When your child or grandma comes to you saying they are hungry, you're going to have to exercise the self-control to tell them "no" and keep them out of the supplies until it's time for the next meal. Yes, it's a hard thing to do, but rationing can offer you some comfort in these troubling circumstances. It ensures that there will be enough to go around for the planned period of time, and in an emergency that is well beyond your control, at least you'll have a sense of control over your own resources.

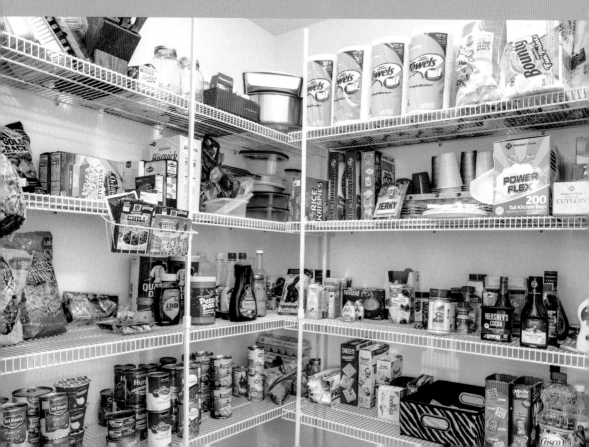

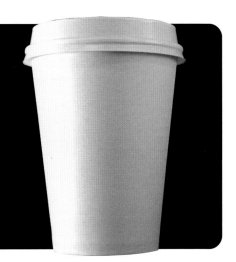

50 BUILD A MENU PLAN

Now that you understand rationing, you can put that wisdom to work by taking an inventory of your food supplies and building a menu plan for a specific number of days. To make this task easier, you don't have to assign specific foods to specific days or meals. A simpler form of emergency food planning is to designate food as either a breakfast food or a lunch/dinner item, and designate those either "fresh" or shelf stable. If you love planning (or are really worried you'll have enough) you can earmark your food in more categories and plan exactly which day you'll have it (but your plan doesn't have to be that detailed).

Here's an example. Let's say that you wanted to ration supplies for the coming week for one person. There is a half of a box of cereal, a pint of milk, a half box of instant oatmeal packets, some random canned goods, and a small amount of meat and veggies in the fridge. It's usually best to use up your fresh food first, to avoid loss from spoilage. So that milk and cereal would be breakfast for the first four days. You'll want to divide the cereal into smaller bags for serving sizes. Split the half of a box of cereal in half, then split the halves in half to get four servings. After the cereal and milk are gone, get into the oatmeal packs for breakfasts. No second breakfasts, just one per day. You can turn the fresh meat and vegetables in the fridge into a soup or stew on day one. One serving would be enjoyed hot, and the leftovers would be divided into separate containers with lids. These would be held for storage in the fridge or freezer, and homemade soup servings could be intermixed with the canned goods for lunches and dinners. As long as you've got a total of fourteen items for lunches and dinners, and seven breakfast items, your week is covered.

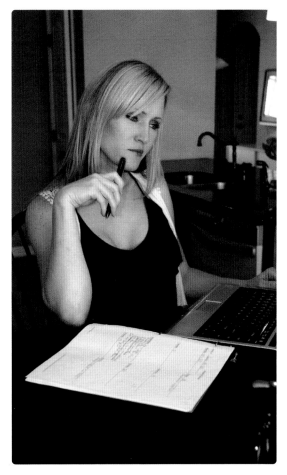

51 KICK A BAD HABIT

Oh no, you're all out of smokes! Or booze. Or whatever else you think you need to live. This could be the perfect occasion to kick a bad habit. With limited access to your vice of choice, you may be able to wean yourself away from the habit forming thing (and rationing comes into play again!). Scale down what you have until you have no "servings" per day. Yes, it's painful. We know. Tim kicked caffeine about eight years ago, and while it was hard, he's so glad he did it since he sleeps much better and wakes up ready to get to work. He found that he didn't "need" it at all. We hope you can all find something that you don't need anymore, to simplify your life and become a healthier person.

52 FIGURE OUT HOW MUCH WATER YOU'LL NEED

Survival guides will tell you to store enough water for a week or more, but how do you know what that means? Look at the figures below, then multiply the daily numbers by 14 for adults, children, elderly, infants, and the sick or wounded to calculate your family's water storage requirements for a two-week emergency.

ACTIVITY LEVEL	BARE BONES	SOME ACTIVITY	DRY CLIMATE OR VERY ACTIVE
ILL, BURNED, OR WOUNDED ADULT	2 GAL (8 L)	3 GAL (11 L)	5 GAL (19 L)
AVERAGE ADULT	1 GAL (4 L)	1.5 GAL (6 L)	3 GAL (11 L)
CHILDREN & ELDERLY	.75 GAL (3 L)	1 GAL (4 L)	2 GAL (8 L)
INFANTS	.5 gal (2 l)	1 GAL (4 L)	2 GAL (8 L)

53 FILL UP!

Water is a top survival priority, and you'll need some on hand, especially if the pandemic is waterborne and the regular water supply is potentially contaminated.

GALLON JUGS Glass wine jugs or juice jugs can be a nice choice for household storage—until you break them. Plastic 1-gallon (4-l) water jugs are more resistant to breakage, but they are vulnerable to leakage and chewing rodents. Don't reuse milk and juice jugs, as they're hard to sanitize and often grow more bacteria.

SODA BOTTLES It's fine to use reclaimed 2-liter soda bottles. Make sure the containers are stamped with HDPE (high-density polyethylene) and coded with the recycle symbol and a number 2 inside. HDPE containers are approved for food and water storage.

WATERBOB This 100-gallon (400-l) water bladder can be laid in a bathtub and filled from the tub's faucet in 20 minutes. It's a great thing to deploy if you know that trouble is coming, such as a hurricane heading for you.

WATER COOLER JUGS The Holy Grail of water containers, the 5-gallon (19-l) jug can hold a lot of water and stay portable. Buy them factory-filled; they'll be safe to drink for a year or more.

55-GALLON (210-L) DRUMS Designed specifically for water storage, these big blue monsters will hold a week's worth of water or more. But they can be difficult to transport if you have to move them when full. Make sure it's a food-grade water barrel. Other barrels may create chemical interactions between the water and the plastic.

54 THINK OUTSIDE THE SINK

While a pandemic may not cause water problems, it can sure as heck slow down how long it takes the city to get things working again if anything does go wrong. If the water stops flowing to your home, you do have a few options to consider before you start sucking on your last ice cubes. There's abundant water hidden in the average dwelling, if you know where to look. Just be sure to treat the water if the pandemic is waterborne.

THE PIPES Even in a utility outage, water can be found lying in the pipes. Open the highest faucet in the house, then open the lowest faucet or spigot, catching the water in some clean containers.

THE HOT WATER HEATER You may find 40 to 80 gallons (150 to 300 l) of drinkable water simply by opening the drain valve at the bottom of the unit and catching the water in a pan or shallow dish. Use this water soon, as the warm water heater is a great bacterial breeding ground. Turn off the power to electric water heaters, as they will burn up with no water in the unit.

THE TOILET TANK To clarify, we are talking about the tank, not the toilet bowl. The tank of every toilet has a gallon (4 l) or more of perfectly clean water in it.

THE FISH TANK A freshwater fish tank can be claimed as a water source, along with koi ponds, fountains, and other water

features. Treat this water with chemicals or by boiling for 10 minutes before drinking.

THE GUTTERS The gutter system on your home can provide many gallons of water from just a light rain shower. Divert your downspouts into rain barrels or other large containers to take advantage of free water from the rainfall.

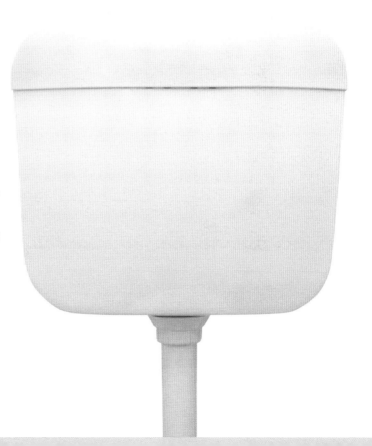

56 STOCK FOOD AND WATER

Even if you're really well prepared, you may end up utilizing tips from the "improvised" set of suggestions as a way of extending your water and food supply in the event of a longer-lasting disaster.

WATER

- Emergency water rations in disaster supplies (5-year shelf life).

- 7-gallon (26.5 liter) water jugs (rotated every six months, and sanitized between uses)

- Filled reusable water bottles in go bags (rotated every 6 months and sanitized between uses)

- Extra cases of coconut water or sports drinks (rotated every year or per expiration date)

FOOD

- Military style MREs in disaster supplies (3- to 5-year shelf life)

- Freeze-dried (20- to 30-year shelf life) and canned goods (1- to 2-year shelf life) stored securely

- Food bars and dried meats (rotated annually or according to expiration date)

- Emergency rations in go bags (rotated annually)

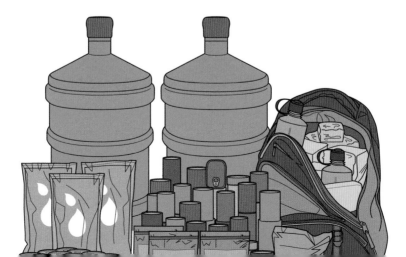

If you haven't been able to put together a proper set of food and water supplies for a disaster, or are in a situation where you can't get to the stocks you have, you can still improvise. Here are some suggestions.

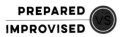
IMPROVISED

FOOD
- Whatever food you have in your fridge and pantry, carefully rationed until help arrives
- Whatever food is available for purchase at stores that might still be open
- Whatever fruits and vegetables might be ripe in your garden

WATER
- Melted ice from freezers
- From the water heater
- From filling bathtub after the disaster (if there is any water pressure available)
- From rain or snow (must be purified before drinking)

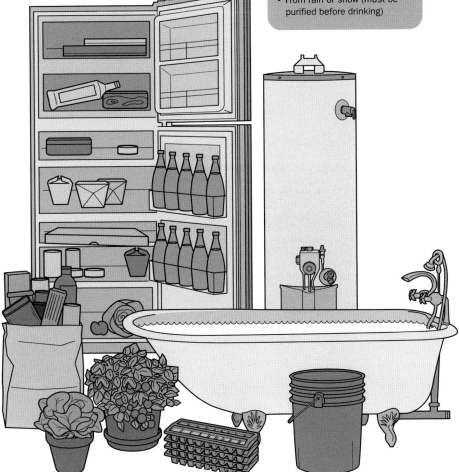

57 FIND THE RIGHT PANTRY SPOT

To get the maximum life span from your stored food, it's critical to store it in a food-friendly location in your home. The traits of a good food storage spot are as follows:

DARK Light can damage many foods and shorten their lifespan.

COOL Low temperatures are critical to storage, and it is best if temps don't fluctuate.

DRY Moisture can allow mold and bacteria to flourish in stored food. Pick a dry spot and package your food to keep moisture out.

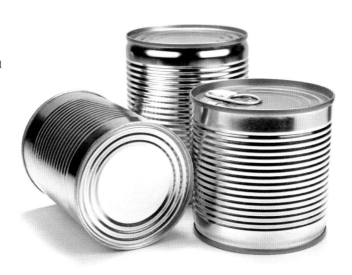

58 CONSIDER EMERGENCY ALTERNATIVES

Emergency supplies should be nonperishable and able to keep for years. Here are the most common options to consider.

FOOD SOURCE	ADVANTAGE	DISADVANTAGE	NOTES
FREEZE DRIED	Very long shelf life	Require water to prepare	Generally considered the best option for taste
CANNED	Inexpensive	Bulky	Problematic in freezing conditions or high humidity (danger of rust)
MRE	Packaged for convenience	Expensive	Taste can be monotonous
DRY GOODS (wheat, rice, corn, sugar, pinto beans, oats, pasta, potato flakes, nonfat powdered milk)	Very long shelf life	Require preparation for storage and usually need other ingredients to cook	Not generally appropriate for shorter-term emergencies
FOOD BARS/JERKY	Portable, easy to eat	Shorter shelf life	Not a satisfying substitute for a meal

59 KEEP CAFFEINE ON HAND

Unless you're trying to kick a coffee habit (see item 54), caffeine can be a vital part of your disaster kit, particularly when it's not easy to prepare coffee or tea. Luckily there are alternatives for a pick-me-up: caffeinated gum and caffeine pills. Neither requires preparation, and they're both compact and easily carried in your go bag, but gum has the added advantage of helping suppress hunger a bit, which may be useful if you're trying to conserve food supplies.

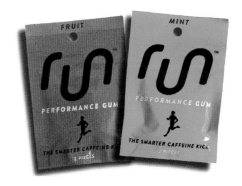

60 TEST YOUR KIT

The only way to know for sure if your emergency supplies (and menu plan) will work for the family is to do a test. This is best done on a long weekend right before rotating supplies that will expire shortly. It's important that everyone in the household understands the need to avoid "cheating" by buying outside food or eating out, as that will likely lead to a false idea of how long your supplies will last. Another reason to test out your supplies? Kids who are stressed or traumatized after a disaster may refuse to eat strange foods, and this gives them a chance to taste everything under normal conditions.

STEP 1 Gather your household and discuss the test, so that everyone can be involved.

STEP 2 Secretly pick a date several months away for the test to happen.

STEP 3 On that date, declare that an "emergency" has happened, and that whatever food and water is in the house is what you have to survive on for the next 5-7 days.

STEP 4 See how long your household can last on your disaster supplies and the available food in your fridge, freezer, and pantry.

STEP 5 Restock disaster supplies and perishable foods.

STEP 6 Enjoy a nice meal in to celebrate.

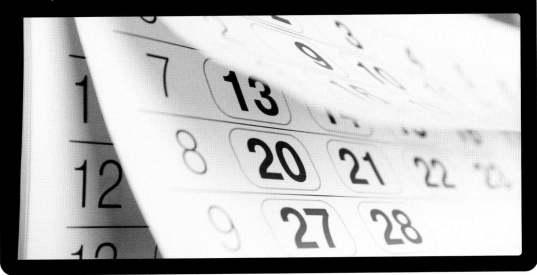

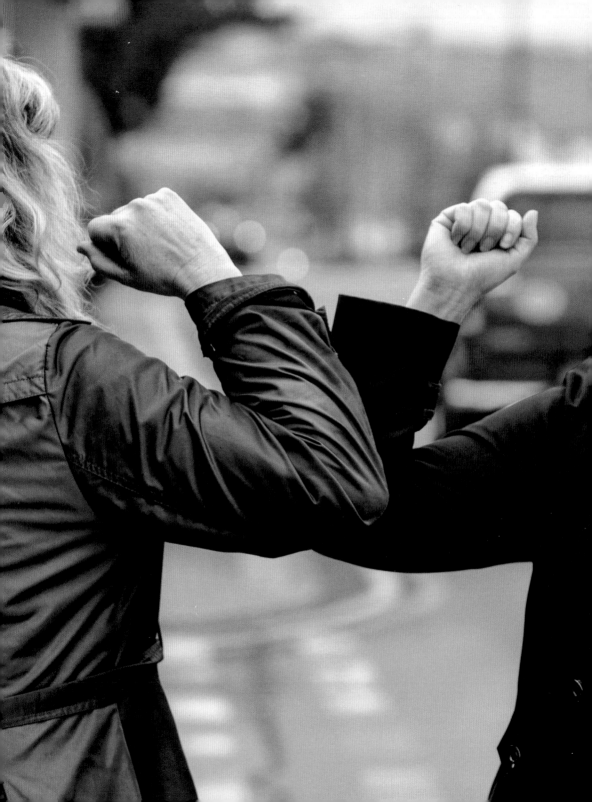

COMMUNITY & FAMILY SUPPORT

There's a certain sort of person who thinks of survival in terms of the Rambo-like rugged individual battling the elements (or terrorists, or giant ants from outer space) alone. That certainly is a form of survival, but it's not the one most of us are most likely to experience.

In fact, if asked, the reality is that most of us would probably rate our family, friends, and pets as the best things in our lives. Knowing how to protect your loved ones in a frightening new situation, and knowing they can count on you, makes all the difference.

MAKE WISE DECISIONS If you're an essential worker, you may not have the option of holing up at home with your loved ones. In that case, change clothes as soon as you get home and shower to keep them safe. In some cases, families have decided to shelter in place together even if that means kids coming home from college and self-quarantining until they're sure of being symptom-free. Do what works for you and your loved ones.

KEEP SPIRITS UP If you can't volunteer in person, find other ways to make human contact. Try an online yoga class or book group, or speak to a therapist over Zoom.

ASK FOR HELP WHEN YOU NEED TO Sometimes one of the most important aspects of being strong is knowing when to take a break, to lean on someone else, to admit that you're scared or overwhelmed. Don't get so caught up in being "the strong one" that you break under the pressure! Your friends and family are there for you.

61 ASSESS AND RESPOND TO AN EMERGENCY

Who is the true hero in an emergency? It's not necessarily the action-star type who comes in swinging— someone who is calm, cool, and collected is much more likely to save the day. Silly as it may sound, practicing strategies to remain calm may very well help. Do you get infuriated when someone cuts you off in traffic? Freak out when the bathtub overflows? Get squeamish at the sight of blood? Instead, take a moment to ask yourself if your reaction is helping to make things better. If not, what would? If you train yourself to handle life's little emergencies, you'll be much better at dealing with life-threatening events.

DON'T PANIC Take an extra moment to breathe deeply and calm yourself before taking any action.

BE REALISTIC Assess what you can realistically do to make a situation better. Prioritize your own health and safety and that of your family.

USE LOGIC Don't think about what you hope you can talk others into doing. What's the best, most logical course of action based on your skills, abilities, and resources? Do that. Worry about everything else later.

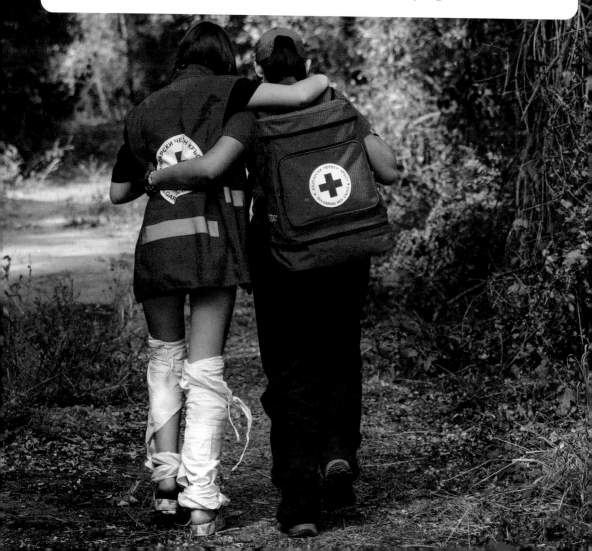

62 SURVIVE ANYTHING

People with no skills and no gear have survived seemingly insurmountable scenarios, simply because they had the right mindset not to become a casualty.

MENTAL TOUGHNESS The strength of your will and the toughness of your mind can trump physical prowess in survival situations. You must learn to tolerate the intolerable, suffer through the insufferable, and overcome your weakness and your desire to give up.

> *Creativity* While other critters use tools and perform complex tasks, they've got nothing on the creativity of the human animal. We are the creature that creates. Over the eons, we've learned how to create fire from sticks and metal from rocks. We turned these things into engines, rockets and computers, and we turned those into the sophisticated modern cultures that we have today. By cultivating our inherent trait of creativity, we can devise unexpected solutions when things get tough. We are descended from some of the smartest people that ever lived, and we were born to be creative.

MOTIVATION What motivates a person to stay alive when everything has gone wrong? Many survival stories speak of the survivor's devotion to a higher power or their intense desire to get back to family, friends, and loved ones. Motivation is the mental aspect that keeps people going beyond all hope or reason.

> *Ignorance* Despite the wealth of information available to the world today, there are a lot of people who couldn't survive even a minor emergency. Most people assume that survival skills are easy because they look easy on TV, and so they overestimate their own abilities. You need to know what to do, how to do it, and you need to have done it before in order to really possess the skills to survive.

ADAPTABILITY The ability to adapt and survival have always been closely related. The ability to adapt to changing events, situations, and environments is one of the most impressive and necessary parts of a survivor's mind-set. You must be able to recognize what's worth continuing and what needs to be abandoned.

> *Stubbornness* This can be a real stumbling block for some people, and it's often confused with tenacity. Don't be afraid to change your mind. If something isn't working, change it up. Don't let your stubborn side get you or someone else killed.

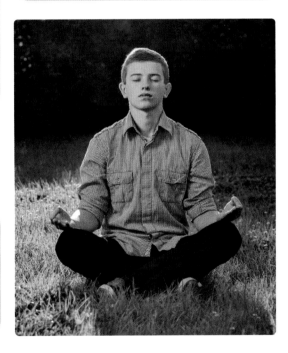

63 DEVELOP AN ATTITUDE

A positive attitude can be a major asset in an emergency. In this case, "positive" doesn't mean "irrationally cheerful" but rather a levelheaded calm with an optimistic spin.

That said, there's room for a more aggressive stance, especially when trouble or danger looms. Of course, we're not suggesting you go berserk on anyone, just noting that a dose of properly harnessed aggression can give you a wellspring of energy in a survival emergency. Get mad. Get mean. When things get ugly, don't just lie down and take it. Kindle that fighting spirit and fight to stay alive

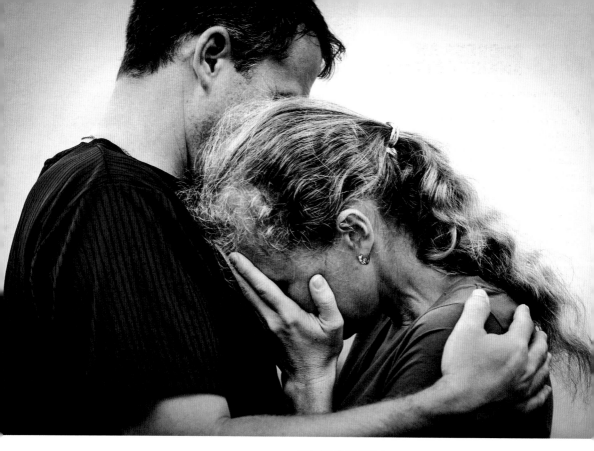

64 UNDERSTAND AND ACCEPT STRESS

Stress is a part of being human. People experience it in a variety of ways in everyday circumstances, at school, at work, and in family life. However, the type of stress you experience during an emergency or large-scale incident can be severe; understanding how it could affect you or others is an important part of self-care and helping others. Everyone who sees or experiences a disaster is affected by it in some way.

It is, for example, normal to feel anxious about your safety and that of your family and friends immediately following an incident. Other normal reactions include a deep sense of sadness, grief, or anger.

Accepting that all of these reactions and feelings are normal can help you to recover more quickly than the people who are lacking this awareness. Integrating the experience can take a long time, sometimes years, and it isn't always easy. Seek the help of mental health professionals or support groups if you feel as if you can't cope on your own.

65 RECOGNIZE SIGNS OF STRESS

People handle stress in many different ways. Even with support and resources, some individuals find themselves unable to cope. Knowing the signs of overwhelming stress can help you decide when to get assistance.

People under significant stress can experience physical reactions including fatigue, unexpected or prolonged cold- or flu-like symptoms, tunnel vision or muffled hearing, headache or stomach problems, or loss of appetite. They may report feeling confused or overwhelmed, with trouble communicating or paying attention. Their emotions may range from sadness, guilt, or frustration to fear, anger, outright denial, or emotional detachment. Conversely, they might also exhibit hyperactivity or hyper-vigilance, have nightmares or trouble sleeping, wild mood swings, or emotional outbursts. They may feel isolated, afraid of crowds or of being alone.

If you observe someone exhibiting these signs, they may need crisis counseling or stress management support.

66 ADDRESS AN ANXIETY ATTACK

Anxiety attacks, also called panic attacks, are episodes of intense panic or fear. They usually occur suddenly and without warning, peak within 10 minutes, and rarely last more than 30 minutes. Shortness of breath and chest pain are sometimes the most significant symptoms; the person may fear incorrectly that they are suffering a heart attack. However, since chest pain and shortness of breath are the hallmark symptoms of cardiovascular illnesses, seeking an emergency medical evaluation is still appropriate to determine the true cause.

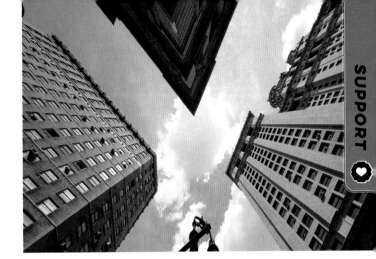

Symptoms of Anxiety Include:

- feeling overwhelmed, detached, or unreal
- feeling like you are losing control or going crazy
- heart palpitations or chest pain
- feeling faint, dizzy, or light-headed
- hyperventilation, trouble breathing, or sensation of choking
- hot flashes or chills (particularly in the facial or neck area)

- trembling or shaking
- nausea or stomach cramps
- numbness or tingling throughout the body
- headache or backache
- sweating
- dry mouth or difficulty swallowing

67 HELP THEM CALM DOWN

Being there for somebody who is experiencing an anxiety attack can really make a big difference to their well-being. Here are some ways to help calm someone under these circumstances.

The person will probably have an overwhelming desire to leave where they are; help them get somewhere quiet and secure. Try to reassure the person repeatedly by letting them know that you're going to help and support them. If you are able to get them into a safe space, reassure them that they are safe.

If the person is having an anxiety attack, get their permission before making physical contact. In some cases, touching without asking can increase the panic and make the situation worse.

Ask the victim what will help them. Sometimes people will know what will help, but may need your assistance to

them, and that if you minimize or dismiss the fear in any way you can make the panic attack worse. Let them talk it out or process their experience, for example, by asking them questions in a calm, neutral way. Listen supportively and accept whatever answer is given.

Help the victim to control their breathing by taking slow, deliberate breaths. Ask them to inhale and exhale on your count. Start off by counting out loud, encouraging the victim to breathe in for 2 seconds and then out for two seconds. After that, gradually increase the count until their breathing has slowed.

Some panic attacks can also be accompanied by sensations of warmth, commonly around the neck and face. A cool, damp cloth can help minimize this sensation and calm the victim.

Stay with the person until they have recovered from

68 TEND TO VICARIOUS TRAUMA

Secondary, or vicarious, stress, can affect people indirectly connected to an incident. Vicarious stress may affect emergency responders and medical professionals, family members who help others and their communities cope with the aftermath, or even those exposed to all the pandemic news coverage. It's important to understand how you or others will be affected in this way, especially since secondary stress manifests in much the same way as those who directly experienced the event. You can use the same stress-management strategies for those who are direct victims of a disaster and to help others who may not realize they are affected since they "weren't there" when it happened.

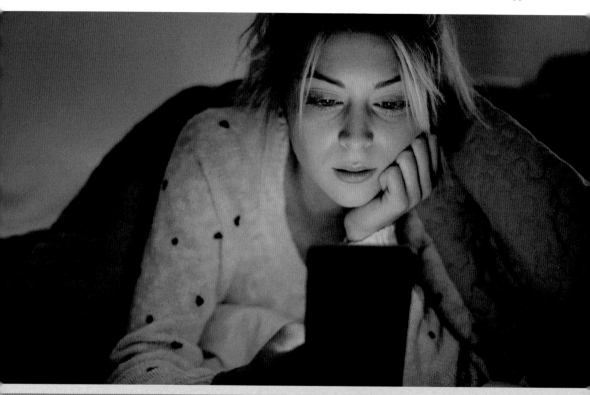

69 MANAGE YOUR MENTAL HEALTH

There are many healthy ways to manage and cope with stress, and to support others in their stress management. You know what's best for you in general, but consider accepting the help offered by community programs and resources . Your family, friends, and religious institutions may also be affected, so get a mix of support from people who are not directly affected as well as from those who can relate. You need to care for your physical, emotional, psychological and spiritual needs.

STAY HEALTHY Get enough sleep, exercise, eat a balanced diet, and find a balance between work and downtime.

CONNECT WITH OTHERS Spend time with family and friends. Be open to receiving as well as giving support. As soon as possible after the incident, reestablish your normal family or daily routine while limiting any demanding responsibilities on yourself and your family.

KEEP YOUR SPIRITS UP Use spiritual resources you have available, and be willing to talk to mental health professionals. Or just talk with someone about your feelings even though it may be difficult. It's important, however, not to force yourself or others to do so.

70 ASK FOR—AND GIVE—HELP

Disasters and emergencies can bring out the best in people—and the worst. Whether you decide to shelter in place or temporarily relocate to a rural area,, you may well need to get some help from others. And others will ask you for assistance. Remember, there is strength in numbers, and you can get more done through cooperation than by going at it alone. But you don't want to be a patsy. Here are some guidelines.

SAY IT RIGHT If you go to your neighbor asking for something during a crisis, you'll probably be rebuffed. But if you go to her offering something, you'll almost always have a warmer reception. Tell the neighbor who you are, that you'd like to help her. Tell her that you're not in charge of anything but you're asking everyone to rally at a certain time and place to discuss the crisis at hand. Get as many neighbors together as you can, and then let nature take its course. Leaders will emerge and plans will form—all because you were the catalyst.

HELP OTHERS, BUT GUARDEDLY Even if you are the biggest prepper hoarder on Earth, you're not going to have enough supplies to take care of everybody. Keep your own safety and security in mind as you help others. No one should know how much food, water, and supplies you have—or where they're located. It's outstanding that you want to help others, and you should. But remember that the person you helped today may be desperate tomorrow—and feeling justified as he or she is taking your stuff by force.

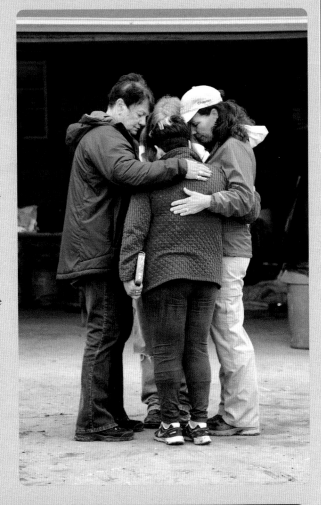

71 SHARE YOUR SKILLS

There are some skill sets that are useful almost anywhere, such as medical training, wilderness survival skills, and so forth. However, you never know what other skills might come in handy. For example, if you're dealing with an epidemic, doctors, nurses, and other medical professionals are obviously crucial. But what if you need to quarantine a group of children in order to keep them safe? A kindergarten teacher would be worth her weight in gold if you needed to keep the youngsters calm and under control. That guy whose hobby is home brewing? He might be able to also make hand sanitizer!

The basic lesson here is that you'll do well if you get to know your neighbors, and encourage everyone to share their skills and interests—whether they seem immediately relevant or not.

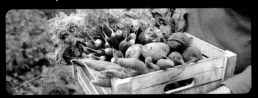

Part of the hard work of parenting involves keeping your kids safe. This hard work is made much harder when we are trying to keep our kids safe during a disaster. Since younger kids can't comprehend the perils of pathogens, their behavior can be tough to modify. For example, many little people love everyone. But in the middle of a pandemic, few things are more terrifying to a parent than having their little one dash down the street to hug a total stranger. Don't be shy when it comes to asking other parents for ideas and support. You'll also want to consider these age-appropriate issues and ways that the kids can help out.

KEEP GRADE SCHOOLERS BUSY If they weren't so cute, we wouldn't be so forgiving with toddlers and elementary-age kids—and their incorrigible difficulty with changes of routine and following new rules. Patience, repetition, and distraction can be the best arrows in a parent's quiver, on an average Tuesday or in the middle of a crisis. Be patient with the kids, since a pandemic will definitely impact the family's routine. Repeat the "new rules" as many times as you need to, until the new information has sunk in. Distract them as needed, with new games, activities and even simple chores, when you need a break to recharge your parental superpower of patience. For example, you can make "picking up" a room into a game, by hiding a snack or surprise under their toys. No, it won't all be fun and games. You may have a hard time explaining to your little one why they can't see grandma (since it raises the idea of grandma being sick), but the extra time you'll spend with your kids can make up some of the difference. Do some things they'll never forget, like howling at the moon every night, and you'll all be able to blow off a little stress (and make some family memories in the process).

GO EASY ON MIDDLE SCHOOLERS This is a tough age for kids in any situation—not little anymore, but not "big kids" in high school either. At this age, the kids are trying to figure out who they are and who they want to be. This is challenging enough, but when we add the challenges of a pandemic to their list of troubles, it can be more than some kids can handle. Like certain teens, middle schoolers may never want to leave their room. Or like younger kids, they may constantly nag you about seeing their friends. As a parent, you'll have to strike a balance between giving them freedom and keeping them on lockdown at home. Good luck with that, as every child is different, and this time of their life is naturally tough for both kid and parent (with the plague knocking on your door). Try to keep them from gaming all day and staying up all night, as they will want to do. This can be easier if you're able to tire them out with supervised

outdoor time. They won't like it, at all, but keep them active with chores around the house as well. Pay them if you must, but find some way to keep them active.

WATCH OUT FOR YOUR TEENS Since they're practically adults, teenagers are old enough to understand the threats they face during a crisis. But they're also still childlike enough to believe they are invulnerable. They will try to sneak out to see their friends, as teens have done for all eternity (especially if you live in the city or suburbs and your teens have neighborhood friends). Do your best to be sure they understand the new rules of a pandemic, and keep a close eye on their social media. Since idle hands are the devil's workshop, keep your tweens and teens busy with things that help the household (like cooking meals) and things that help the community (like sewing masks, putting together donations for the less fortunate, and so forth). They're not babies anymore, but until they fly the nest, try your best to watch over them and keep them busy.

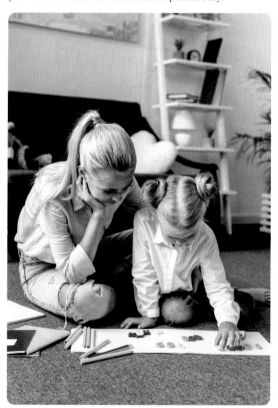

73 PITCH IN AS A FAMILY

Helping kids prepare for emergencies can be scary for them. But assuring kids that planning and preparing allows everyone to better handle the problem can help them cope. Here are some age-appropriate activities to help kids prepare for pandemics and other scary situations.

ELEMENTARY SCHOOL AGE

- Conduct a scavenger hunt for items that should go into an emergency kit.
- Volunteer to take part in a food drive or other community preparedness activity.
- Discuss different places where emergencies could happen (such as at school, at home, or at a park) and how to prepare for those different types of situations.
- Have children write and illustrate a storybook on how to prepare for an emergency.
- Ask them questions such as: What do we do when a tornado comes? What is an emergency plan? Where is our emergency kit? What do we put into it?
- Work together to make a mini disaster kit and go bag for each child; include a few fun toys and something else that provides them comfort, like a stuffed animal.

MIDDLE SCHOOL / JUNIOR HIGH

- Take a first-aid or CPR class.
- Teach them how to shut off the utilities in case of emergency.
- Have them write a report, create a poster, or make a short video about a specific hazard.
- Tour a fire department or other emergency service provider.
- Take a class to get licensed for HAM radio.
- Work together to create an everyday carry kit.

HIGH SCHOOL AGE

- Volunteer with the Red Cross, a local CERT (Community Emergency Response Team) program, or a fire department explorer program.
- Create an emergency kit for their car.
- Have them write an article for their school newspaper or blog or do a school assignment on emergency preparedness.
- Brainstorm how they could work with a local disaster relief organization to prepare others for an emergency, and then make it happen.
- Teach them how to purify water with bleach, by boiling, or with other water-purification techniques.

74 BE HONEST WITH KIDS

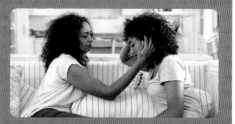

As a parent you want to protect your children during a disaster. You may not want to discuss the situation in front of them, or let them see how worried you are, but avoiding the issue might be equally stressful for them. Listen to your kids and ask them about their feelings. Give an appropriate amount of detail for them to understand the situation.

KNOW YOUR KIDS Keep in mind that most kids possess an endearing blend of naivety and skepticism. For example, they may believe in Santa Claus wholeheartedly, while in seemingly stark contrast, also having an internal "lie detector" that can be alarmingly accurate, catching their parents in the slightest alteration of the truth when it's least convenient.

TELL TOUGH TRUTHS Don't try to sugar-coat the truth or attempt to minimize the scope of what's happening in a pandemic. Chances are good that they'll know you're lying. Tell them the truth, as much as someone of their age group can handle and keep them updated as you see fit. It's probably a good idea to limit (or eliminate) their exposure to the 24-hour disaster news channel, since the gloom-and-doom coverage can weigh heavily on their young minds. Let them hear the facts from you, and shoot straight with them.

EXPLAIN CLEARLY Explain the issues at hand and share the details of your plan to get through it. Pick your words carefully and explain that while this disease is bad, if our whole family follows the rules, we should be fine. Remind them that even if one of the family members becomes ill, almost everyone who gets COVID-19 does actually make a full recovery.

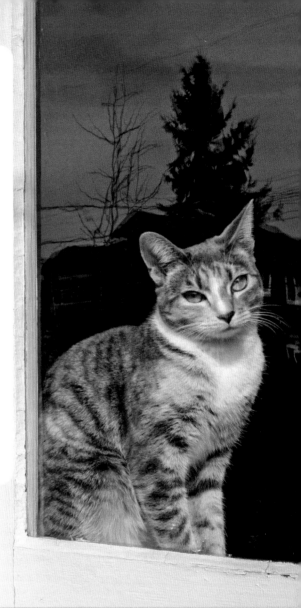

75 DON'T FORGET YOUR PETS

During times of crisis, pets often become separated from their owners. Some of the most heartwarming reunion tales in post-disaster areas are the unexpected, less-than-likely ones between pets and their long-lost owners. Unfortunately, there's a reason these are so touching—because they're surprising. More often than not, upheaval will separate you from a furry friend for good—but here are a few ways to make sure that you can find your way back to your little survivor.

MICROCHIPPING Microchip implants are permanent, inexpensive, and very common, so shelters and veterinarians know to check for them. You can change the associated information if you move or your phone number changes—just call up the company to make sure it's up to date.

DIGITAL ID TAGS Sure, Fido can have the regular kind on his collar—but a digital QR code can be updated more easily than an engraving. There are also special collars with USB clips, so your pet is always carrying around a handy emergency flash drive with your info.

DUCT TAPE Yet another use for our favorite supply-kit item: If your pet has the old-fashioned tags, write your new information and where you are traveling on a strip of duct tape, and attach it to the back of the tag.

76 QUARANTINE WITH FIDO AND FLUFFY

So, you're sheltering in place with your pets and maybe you're trying to work from home, study, or doing home improvement projects to pass the time since you're stuck indoors. Your pets don't know why you're home all the time, they are just glad that you're there more, so you must be available to pet them and play with them more, right? They are like little kids in that way, but you can plan ahead for their needs too, and keep some extra toys and treats in your disaster kit so you can keep them distracted when they want all of your attention. This is especially true of pets that normally are allowed to go in and out as they please, remember their world just got a lot smaller and they will get bored. So it's either new toys and more playtime, or they will make something you care about, like your favorite shoes, into their next toy.

77 KEEP EACH OTHER HEALTHY

Whenever a new disease surfaces, one of the first questions is always, is there a danger I might get it from my pet? Or that I might give it to them? The short answer is, it depends on the disease pathogen. If you're not sure the best approach to protect you and your pets during a pandemic is to assume that pets can infect humans, and humans can infect pets. So when you're out for a walk apply the same social distancing guidelines you would use for a person to the dogs and other pets you might meet along the way. Don't let other dogs that are not part of your household play with or sniff your dogs. Also, don't let others pet your dogs and don't pet other animals. Essentially, protect them as you would any other member of your household. For many this is easy because they already love and treat your pets like family. If you have a dog that mostly lives outside, or if you have cats that you normally allow to go outside, now would be a great time to consider making them indoor only pets, except for when you take them out on walks. Not only does that protect your pets, but it also provides you with a great source of stress relief and comfort. If you spend just 90 seconds petting an animal you love, your blood pressure goes down an average of 15 systolic, and given that pandemics are stressful, this is good for your health. That said, if you pet becomes sick during a pandemic, take them to the vet and apply the same pandemic precautions as you would with any other person, such as thoroughly washing your hands after touching them and not letting them lick your face.

78 TRAIN FOR DISASTER

Training your pet is a very important part of an easy getaway and for keeping it out of harm's way. It's unsafe to let your pet roam loose when there may be hazards or disorienting scents or other stimuli nearby, so keep it leashed (even if it normally comes when called), and do some crate training.

- Use an airline-approved crate, which most pet-friendly hotels also accept as standard.
- It should be large enough that your pet has 2–3 inches (5–8 cm) of clearance when standing up completely and enough room to turn around.
- When training, introduce the crate gradually. Position it somewhere your pet likes to be, and put a favorite toy inside.
- If your pet is hesitant, take apart the crate and remove the top and door. Allow your pet to go freely in and out of the open half until putting the top back on doesn't cause alarm.

79 STOCK A PET EMERGENCY KIT

If you might need to evacuate with your pet, be sure you're ready to go. Have a bag packed ready with these essentials.

- Pet food in airtight containers
- Registration, rabies, and vaccination records (very important for shelters)
- Necessary pet meds
- Water
- Collar with ID tags
- Sturdy leash or harness
- Travel carrier or crate
- Cat litter and box, doggy clean-up baggies
- Photo IDs of you and your pet
- Cleaning and deodorizing materials
- Familiar items (toys, blankets)
- First-aid supplies (an eyedropper and syringe is useful for administering meds or flushing wounds, and hydrogen peroxide will disinfect as well as induce vomiting in case of poison ingestion)

80 IF YOU MUST GO

If you absolutely have to leave your pet behind, and there is even the smallest chance you might not be able to make it back, there are some important steps to take. Place your pet inside an interior room (or rooms, with interior doors propped open so they can't shut themselves in one area) for safety, and consider leaving a TV or radio on to distract from outside sounds. Leave plenty of food and water in non-spillable bowls. You can also remove the toilet seats and fill the bathtubs with water for them to drink. Last, place signs on exterior doors to alert rescuers, and write your contact info on your pet's crate, then leave it just inside the door.

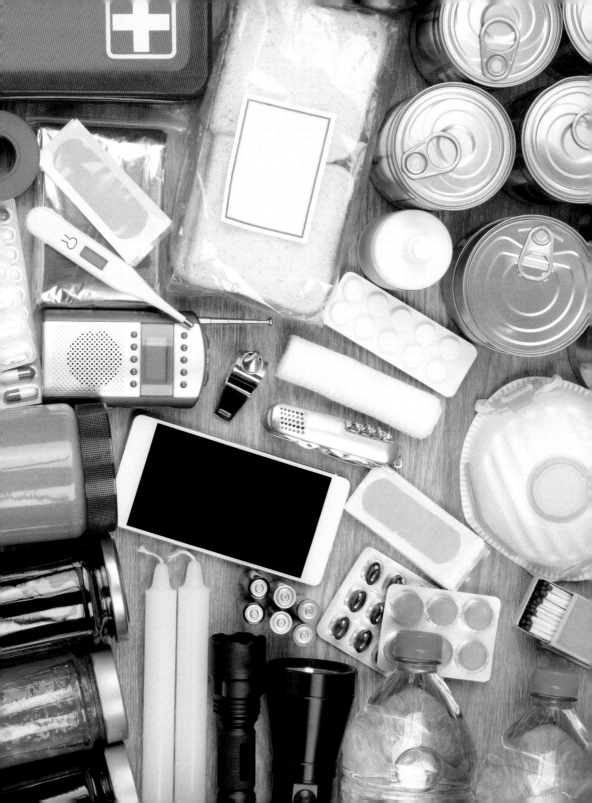

PLAN FOR IT

BE READY FOR THE NEXT EMERGENCY

Every so often, one of us makes an absolutely spot-on prediction and gets the momentary joy of saying "I told you so" to everyone who doubted us. Those predictions? Some of us are better informed than others, but nobody's right 100% of the time about anything.

All of that said, you don't need Madame Cleo's crystal ball to predict that the future will disasters and emergencies for all of us. And fortune will always favor the prepared.

FUTURE PANDEMICS We can certainly take some comfort from the fact that this coronavirus is the first global contagion since the flu of 1918. And if we're very lucky, we'll get another hundred years until something else this bad. But even a less deadly outbreak can cause a lot of suffering, and these preparations are good practice regardless.

BE INFORMED As the cliche would have it, knowledge is power. Knowledge backed up with training, safety drills, and a pantry full of shelf-stable meals is a whole lot more powerful. This chapter is filled with information on staying in touch and connected no matter what.

DISASTERS HAPPEN Perhaps you're reading this book as part of thinking ahead to the next pandemic, or maybe you live in tornado alley or earthquake country and want to be sure you're ready for whatever the future may bring. Read up on your options and talk with your family about a preparedness plan that meets your needs.

81 CREATE AN EMERGENCY PLAN

Now that you've built a disaster readiness kit, you need an emergency plan. In the event of a crisis, a well-thought-out family emergency plan can eliminate stress, limit confusion, and save a great deal of time. Instead of wasting precious minutes wondering what to do or when to do it, you can put your emergency plan to work right away, bringing sanity and safety to dangerous situations. Your family's emergency plan should encompass the following.

- Maintaining up-to-date contact information cards or sheets for each family member

- Communication strategies for keeping in touch, with options in case the phones are out

- Ways to assist or care for anyone with mobility or medical issues, communication difficulties, or special needs.

- The maintenance, inspection, and rotation of emergency supplies, such as non-perishable food, water, first aid, etc. lighting, and communication equipment

- The maintenance of specialized supplies for any infants, young children, or elderly in your family

- A plan and supplies for the care of pets and livestock

- The knowledge and tools to shut off your utilities

- Self-sufficiency skills and supplies, should you have to shelter in place without utilities

- Evacuation plans and routes, should you have to leave your home

- Learn and practice skills such as first aid and CPR.

82 PLAN WISELY

One important part of planning for emergencies is determining which disasters are most likely to affect your household. The most common group is natural disasters, which affect hundreds of thousands of people every year worldwide. You probably don't have to worry much about hurricanes in the Midwest or blizzards in the Caribbean. Many disasters are predictable events, but others, unfortunately, can hit us by surprise.

Common natural disasters can include tornadoes, hurricanes, severe thunderstorms, wild fires, winter storms, earthquakes, and extreme heat. Extreme heat and drought have killed more people in the U.S. since 1970 than any other natural disaster, though they were followed closely by fatalities from flooding and severe thunderstorms. The threat of pandemics or other illness have increased as well. And finally, the threat of a disaster spawned from terrorism has caused many people to take emergency preparedness into their own hands.

83 PUT ACTION IN YOUR PLAN

Counting water bottles and inspecting batteries aren't the only things you'll want to do for emergency planning. You and your family will need to be prepared to act—especially on short notice. Get every family member involved!

GET THE LAY OF THE LAND Draw a map of your home and every potential escape route.

PLAN A MEETING PLACE Determine a meeting place near your home, if your family needs to rally outside of the house.

GO FURTHER ABROAD Pick a meeting place outside of your neighborhood, to be used if you cannot return home or are told to evacuate.

LOOK AT THE ROUTES Decide which route you'd take to get to meeting places, plus an alternate route in case the first is unusable.

CHOOSE A CONTACT
Pick a contact person outside of your immediate area who could relay messages if your household is separated or unable to communicate with each other.

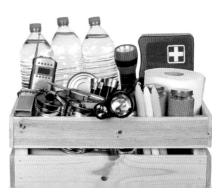

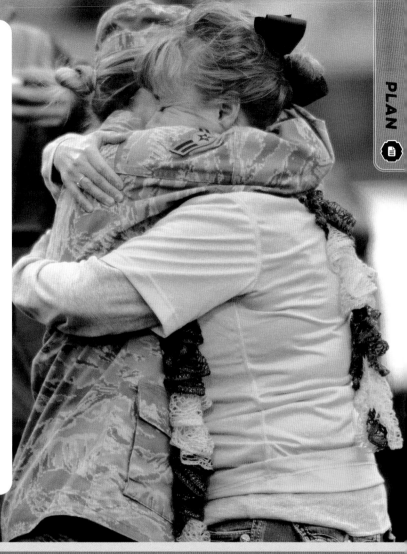

84 KEEP IN CONTACT

It's important that everyone in your household knows the plan for getting in touch with everyone else after a disaster. Even if you've loaded all the information into your mobile phones, consider also keeping a paper copy in case your phone is dead when you need the information.

Include the contact information for each member of your household; make sure that it lists their full name, relation to the family, work and/or school address and phone number, mobile phone number, their e-mail address, and any other contact info that might be relevant.

Don't forget to include important information, such as date of birth, medical insurance policy, blood type, allergies, or medical conditions. Also add names and contact information for any designated out-of-town family contacts.

List muster or evacuation points from your family plan. Review and update the information in the plan annually. Additionally, ensure all members of your household have ICE entries or the emergency contact function active on their phones.

85 COMMUNICATE IN A DISASTER

During a regional emergency or disaster, mobile phone systems quickly become overloaded with voice calls. If you cannot get through, try text messaging instead, as that has a much higher chance of getting through during those circumstances.

If you want to communicate to everyone easily with a single step, consider posting to Twitter, Facebook, or other social media with your status. Alternatively, the Red Cross offers a free "Safe and Well" online listing service. Just be sure to plan with other members of your household which of these systems you'll use should you not be reachable by phone.

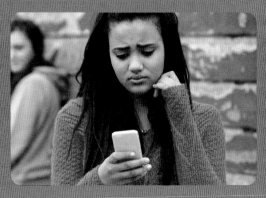

86
COMMUNICATE CLEARLY

In an extended power outage or other disaster, it's likely that your landline, cell phone, or Internet connection will stop working. Here are some items you can use to keep you safe and communicating with others.

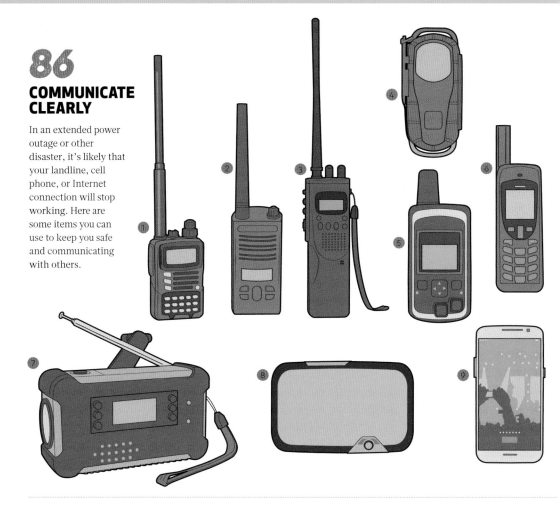

1 HAM RADIO Amateur radio might seem almost quaint, but during a disaster, HAM radio is often one of the most reliable ways to communicate with others and call for help. Handheld radios have a limited range, however, a network of free repeaters can extend coverage over hundreds of miles, and base stations with large antennas can communicate globally, but you'll need to get a license.

2 MURS RADIO Multi-Use Radio Service (MURS) is the big brother to the inexpensive Family Radio Service (FRS) devices in common use today on ski slopes and camping trips. Both types are license-free, but MURS has

better range and is less crowded with other users. Neither radio type has a formal emergency channel; however, they can provide easy and inexpensive communication for neighborhood watch and other groups.

3 CITIZEN'S BAND RADIO CB radios have a highly dedicated following even though the older technology suffers from poorer audio quality than its modern cousins, the handheld range is relatively small, and the units tend to be bulky. However, CB channel 9 is a monitored emergency channel that can be used to call for help, which makes CB still relevant in areas with no cell coverage.

4 PERSONAL LOCATOR BEACONS PLBs have their origins in maritime and aviation search and rescue. Once modern electronics decreased the size of a unit to that of a large cell phone, it was possible for portable applications like hiking or backcountry skiing to make use of the technology. By combining a radio transmitter and GPS receiver, a PLB first sends a unique code that identifies you and then broadcasts a homing signal to allow planes to find your location. You may be billed for the cost of your rescue.

5 SATELLITE MESSENGERS Using the same technology and network

DEVICE	TYPICAL COST	MONTHLY FEES	LICENCE REQUIRED[1]	DEPENDABLE AVERAGE RANGE (MILES)	POWER (WATTS)	VOICE/TEXT/DATA
HAM (UHF)	$200–300	None	Yes	3[1]	5	Yes/No/Yes[2]
MURS	$100–200	None	No	2	2	Yes/No/No
GMRS	$50	None	Yes	1	5	Yes/No/No
FRS	$25	None	No	<1	0.5	Yes/No/No
CB	$100	None	No	2	5	Yes/No/No
PLB	$150–300	None	No	Global	N/A	No/No/No
SATELLITE PHONE	$200–1000	Yes	No	Global	N/A	Yes/Yes/Yes
SATELLITE MESSENGER	$200–300	Yes	No	Global	N/A	No/Yes/Yes
BLUETOOTH MESSAGING	Free	None	No	200 feet	N/A	No/Yes/Yes

[1] Can be extended to hundreds of miles/km with repeaters.   [2] Requires additional hardware.

as satellite phones, these compact devices are used similarly to a PLB to call for help, send text messages, and transmit their location so others can track the user on a website. They are popular with hikers and long-distance travelers who don't need the function or expense of a full satellite phone.

6 SATELLITE PHONE The per-minute cost of a satellite call is much higher than that of a regular cell phone—but worth it in an emergency. Intended for areas where there is no cell phone coverage, they're also extremely helpful when a disaster affects the local phone infrastructure. If you need one temporarily, plenty of companies rent them for short-term use.

7 HAND-CRANKED RADIO No longer just a type of AM/FM/weather radio, these handy devices are also a functional hub with multiple charging options (including AC, DC, battery, solar, and USB), a flashlight, a USB port for charging small electronics, audio jacks for use as an external speaker, and a versatile part of every home disaster kit.

8 WIRELESS HOTSPOTS These are useful in everyday settings, but when your Internet connection is lost due to infrastructure damage, it can take awhile to get back online. If you absolutely need to be online, one of these devices will provide you with

Internet access anywhere there is a 4G connection available.

9 BLUETOOTH MESSAGING APP The newest classification of instant messenger apps, such as FireChat for smartphones, uses bluetooth technology instead of an Internet connection or mobile phone coverage. This allows the phone to be used anywhere, even if networks are down, in a peer-to-peer mode that also helps you discover who is nearby. Coordinate with others in advance so that everyone in a group has the app downloaded before you lose network connectivity for any reason.

87 KNOW THE PLAN

Places where communities commonly gather, work, and play often develop their own emergency and disaster plans. If you or your family spend time at any of these facilities, especially as a student, employee, or volunteer, take the time to learn about what plans are in place. Some entities will provide this information on their website, but others may require attending meetings or inquiring directly. By informing yourself, you can better plan for how you or a member of your family might be affected by a disaster or an emergency based on where they might be at the time.

Consider looking into the disaster plans of places that you frequent, such as schools, workplaces, churches, day-care centers, and neighborhood associations, as well as stadiums, recreation areas, municipalities, and counties.

Additionally, if you live near one of these facilities, being informed about how their emergency response may affect you can help you plan ahead, and they may have additional resources available to you if they have been structured as a community disaster partner.

If you're not sure what to ask or look for in a plan, here are some good starting questions:

- What hazards, emergencies, or disasters are included?
- How are alerts and warnings issued?
- How often are plans updated, and is there a public review process to provide input?
- What are the local considerations for sheltering-in-place and evacuating?
- What else does the plan contain?
- Are plans available for download or review?
- Are there ways to learn more about preparedness?

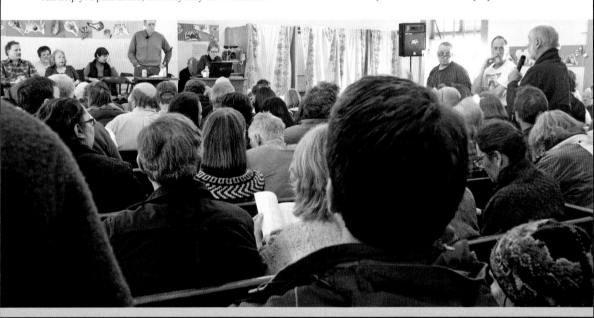

88 BE A COMMUNITY ACTIVIST

If there is no plan in an organization, consider appealing to its leadership to create a plan. Also, consider asking how to get involved in the planning process. Plans for disasters are best made when there is input and involvement from various stakeholders. If your initial efforts to set up a communal planning process fail, turn to other members of your local community and encourage them to voice their concerns. Last, you can contact politicians, local news media, or social media to raise awareness and concern. Since the goal is to create a resilient community, if you reach out to others, this is a good way to find common ground and build consensus and collaboration.

89 LEND A HELPING HAND

Volunteering is a great way to contribute to your community in a time of need, but it can also provide you the opportunity to learn some new skills, get access to training, and practice so that when you need to use those skills you'll be better prepared. Here are a few varieties of volunteer organizations and some of the skills you can learn from being involved.

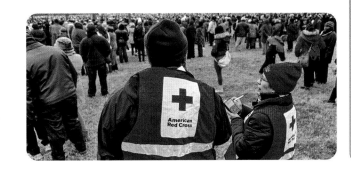

ORGANIZATION	LEARNING OPPORTUNITIES
AMATEUR RADIO EMERGENCY SERVICE (ARES)	HAM radio, emergency communications
CIVIL AIR PATROL (CAP)	Search and rescue, disaster relief
COMMUNITY EMERGENCY RESPONSE TEAM (CERT)	Light search and rescue, incident command, first aid, triage, fire safety, emergency response
NATIONAL WEATHER SERVICE (SKYWARN)	Storm spotting, severe weather assistance
RADIO AMATEUR CIVIL EMERGENCY SERVICE (RACES)	HAM radio, emergency communications
RED CROSS	Disaster response, first aid, shelter operations
SEARCH AND RESCUE (SAR)	Search and rescue, incident command

90 GET EDUCATED

You can learn basic first aid from books and smartphone apps, but proper training is still best. Courses are available from various organizations; check the Red Cross, your local fire department, junior colleges, and community centers. Your next question is: "What classes should I take?" That will depend on your free time, personal interest, and needs.

Ideally you should have advanced first aid, CPR, and AED (automated external defibrillator) training. If you're short on time, a regular first aid class and an abbreviated hands-only CPR class is a good alternative. If you have pets, a pet first aid class may help you get your four-legged friends through times when you can't get to a vet clinic.

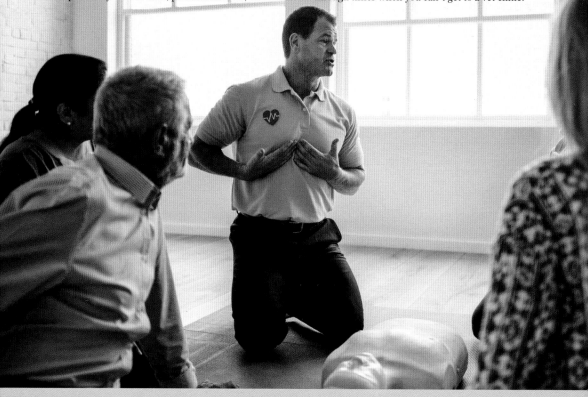

91 GET SOME SERIOUS TRAINING

If you want to dive deep into medical training, here are a few choices, each of which will give you a different set of tools.

BE A FIRST RESPONDER Emergency medical response (EMR) training is the shortest and easiest to complete. It's useful for those who want to focus on immediate emergencies, in support of emergency medical services (EMS) in disasters or smaller events.

GET TECHNICAL Emergency medical technician (EMT) courses are more comprehensive, focusing on geriatric

issues, ambulance operations, and equipment you're unlikely to have in your home. This course is more applicable to those interested in volunteering with EMS or having a broad set of skills past immediate first aid.

GO WILD Wilderness EMT training is a great option for those who go camping, hiking, or otherwise spend lots of time in remote wilderness. The skills learned in this class emphasize improvising and helping others with a minimum of resources. However, this class is the most time consuming.

92 HELP THEM FEEL SAFE

Regardless of training, one of the most important skills to use, whether treating someone who has a minor scrape or a life-threatening injury, is to help make them feel comforted and safe. But this isn't a technique you'll learn in a first-aid class. It's about approaching an injured person as one human who cares about another. Injured patients are often scared and confused, sometimes in ways that are not immediately obvious.

Reassuring your patient is simple: Tell them that they are safe, that you are there to help them, and that responders are on the way. It may also help to explain what's happening around and to them. You might have to overstate the obvious, but if a patient is in shock, they might be overwhelmed by events. Your calm narration will reduce their anxiety, and their experience of the trauma can be more easily handled. It's one of those moments when you really get to be the hero that makes the difference.

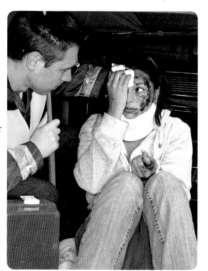

Focus on using positive statements that are true and applicable to the circumstances. For example, somebody who is trapped under a beam after an earthquake is hard to reassure when you don't know how soon responders will get there or when the next aftershock will happen. Circumstances can be challenging, and doing your best will go a long way to helping the person know that they are in good hands.

93 CHECK FOR AN ALERT

If you come across somebody who is unconscious or no longer can speak due to a possible allergic reaction, take a moment to check for a medical alert bracelet, necklace, or, less common, key-chain, wallet card, or kid's shoe tag. The reverse side of the tag will have basic information such as his or her name, emergency contact, and critical medical information including allergies, medications, advance medical directives, and medical conditions such as epilepsy, diabetes, or asthma.

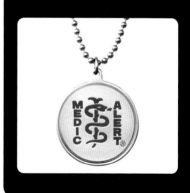

94 TAKE IT TO THE NEXT LEVEL

If you've taken the classes described in this chapter, or just have a desire to be even more helpful in a crisis, you might want to add the following items to your stash of medical supplies. If you look for what's called a "jump bag," you'll find that they often come prepacked with these items—and much more!

- BloodStopper bandages
- Chemical cold packs
- Normal saline (for rinsing injuries)
- Tourniquet
- Stethoscope
- Oral glucose tablets (for diabetic emergencies)
- QuikClot (for controlling bleeding)
- Oropharyngeal (OPA) airway kit
- Penlight
- Activated charcoal (for ingested poisons)
- Blood pressure cuff

95 MAKE A DATE TO PREPARE

If you find the idea of comprehensive disaster preparedness too overwhelming or time-consuming, an easy way to make it manageable is to space the different tasks throughout the year so that everything gets done and checked annually. On the first of each month, check this handy calendar and schedule the month's activities with your family.

MONTH	CATEGORY	KEY TASK	REVIEW
JANUARY	COMMUNICATION PLAN	Discuss and create plans with your household	Review plans with everyone in the household
FEBRUARY	WATER SUPPLY	Review normal water supply, create a 5 to 7 day disaster supply	Replace water supply as needed
MARCH	FOOD SUPPLY	Review pantry, establish a 5 to 7 day disaster food supply	Replace food supply as needed
APRIL	EVACUATION ROUTES	Determine two escape routes from your house and the region	Review plans with everyone in the household
MAY	FIRST AID KIT	Gather necessary supplies	Review kit; replace used supplies; add other supplies if needed
JUNE	DOCUMENTS AND KEYS	Make copies of important documents and keys	Review keys and documents; update or replace if needed
JULY	EQUIPMENT AND TOOLS	Check current setup; purchase any needed items to complete the kit	Replace any missing items
AUGUST	SANITATION AND HYGIENE	Gather supplies in a large waterproof container	Replace any expired items
SEPTEMBER	MEDICINE KIT	Review everyone's prescription needs; create a disaster backup supply	Rotate the backup supply before medications expire
OCTOBER	CLOTHING AND BEDDING	Pack clothing (options for warm, wet, and cold weather) and bedding for each person	Ensure clothes still fit; inspect for damage and wash items if needed
NOVEMBER	HOME HAZARDS	Identify hazards in and outside home; mitigate if possible	Review existing hazards; search for new ones
DECEMBER	PET EMERGENCY SUPPLIES	Establish a 5 to 7 day food supply	Replace supplies and food as needed

96 BACK UP YOUR PLANS

Regardless of whether you're creating emergency plans, stockpiling supplies, selecting equipment, or learning skills, you should have layers of redundancy just in case something fails. This means that when you're making plans, you should also design a plan B whenever reasonably possible. If there are other obvious options, consider coming up with multiple backup plans. It's impossible to plan for every contingency, but having several preplanned options can make the stress of an emergency easier to deal with, provided the plans are not so detailed as to burden you in the moment. You should also look at other resources in this way. Having multiple ways to treat water to make it safe to drink isn't just prudent; it may mean the difference between survival and tragedy. Skills should ideally not have a single point of failure either, so get yourself—and your loved ones—trained in first aid and other needed life-safety skills. In the end, as the famous Franz Kafka quote goes, it's "better to have, and not need, than to need, and not have."

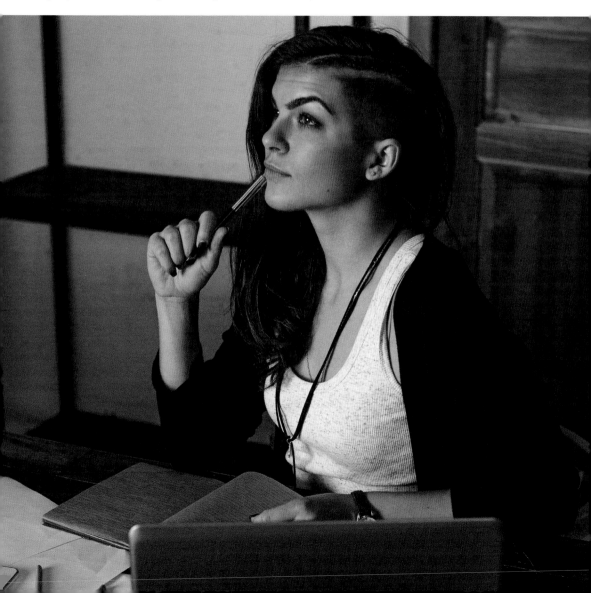

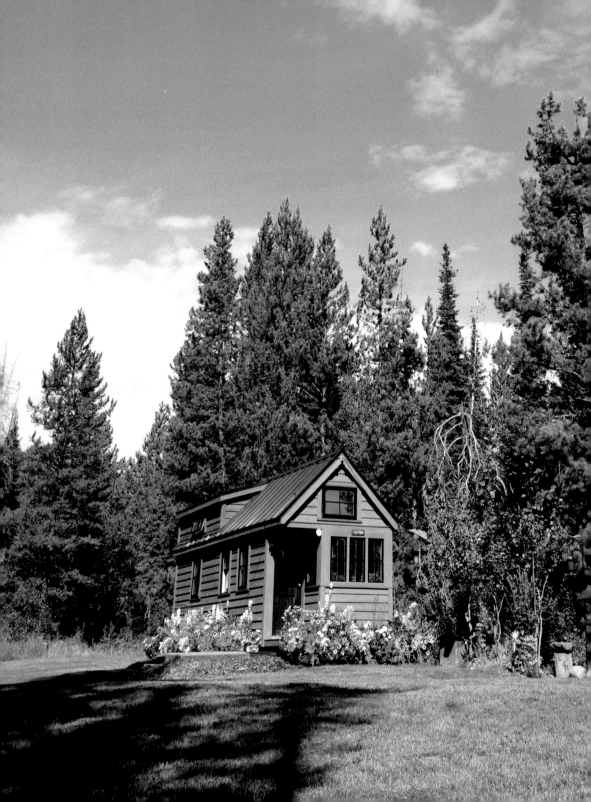

GET OFF THE GRID

There's a silver lining in most disasters, and our hope is that you'll be inspired to become more self-reliant and independent. Who knows, you may even develop a taste for solitude, even after life returns to normal.

Self-sufficiency can manifest itself in many ways, such as growing your first vegetable garden or building a long-term food storage reserve. The drive to provide for yourself may even lead you to make big changes (like moving off the grid, where no one can cough on you). Whole books have been written on the topic (shameless self-promotion: Check out "Recommended Reading" at the back of this book for a few we think are pretty darn cool), but here are some absolute basics you'll want to consider as you ponder this option.

SORT OUT POWER AND WATER Two of the cornerstones of living off the grid are power and water. Here, we'll provide you with a few easy options to provide these for your home. Without these vital resources, no homestead will last very long.

BUILD YOUR FOOD SECURITY It takes time to grow crops and raise livestock, but with a supply of canned and dried food, you'll always have something to eat. Careful planning and taking advantage of bulk foods can give you a diverse diet at a bargain price.

GROW YOUR OWN For those dedicated to self-reliance, growing your own food and medicine can provide many benefits. Not only can you resupply with fresh food and medicine when your stocks run low, you can reduce your trips to the store.

97 MAKE A PLAN

So, you've decided to take the plunge, and make your off-the-grid dream a reality. What next? Before you spend a single dime on land, lumber, or livestock, think long and hard about the difference between your wants and your needs. For example, if you're living in a crowded city, you may want to find your own pristine parcel of land without another neighbor at all for miles around. But just how remote do you need to be in order to be at peace and off the grid? If it takes you a three-day walk to reach the nearest town, this might be a bit too much for a recent urbanite. A common knee-jerk reaction when fleeing from an unhappy situation is to go to extremes, but do you really need to isolate yourself from the world to be happy? For most people, the right location will lie somewhere in between the city and the wilderness. The real trick is finding a good balancing point between a happy, comfortable, modern life, and a romanticized back-to-the-land fantasy that can turn out to be too much work for you to sustain.

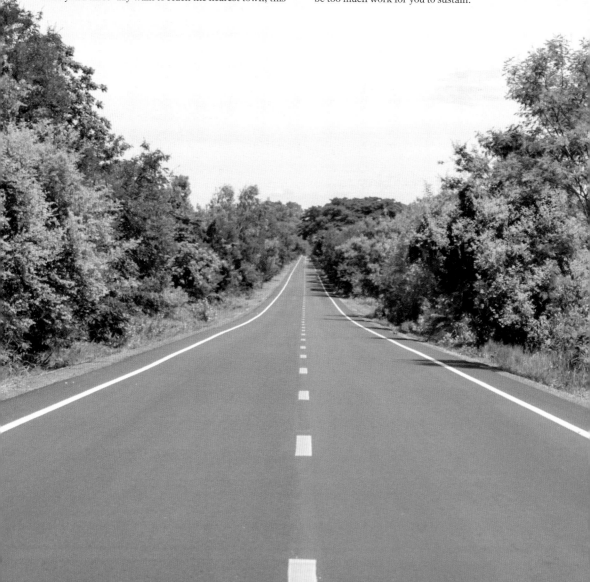

98 GET THE LAY OF THE LAND

All the hard work in the world may not turn a terrible site into the bastion of self-sufficiency you deserve and desire. This is why it's so important to look at all of the good points and the bad ones of a land parcel when searching for the site of your off-grid oasis.

WATER Ideally, the land should have some manner of water source on it, such as a stream, pond, river frontage, or even a boggy area that could be excavated and turned into a clear pond. Find out (if you can) whether the water on the site is seasonal or is present year-round.

OPEN SKY Look for land with about 50 percent open sky and 50 percent wooded. This can give you the best of both worlds. In the northern hemisphere, look for sites with open southern exposure for both solar power and gardening.

ACCESS AND LIMITATIONS Find out about all of the local laws that impact your use of the property. Can you even build anything there or put a road on it? Is the road maintained by the state up to your property? Do you have to take care of the road yourself with the assistance of your neighbors? What about zoning for agricultural use? Do you need building permits for anything besides the home? Will you have to travel over an easement to get to your land? If you will be planning to raise critters, are you allowed to have the ones you want? Yes, this is a lot of questions, and there are many more you should ask. The point is to do the research before it's too late, so that nothing catches you by surprise.

WEATHER The weather will be greatly impacted by the geographic region you choose, but local features (such as mountains) can also create their own micro-climates. Try your best to get an idea of the average rainfall numbers, high and low temperatures, wind and storms, and so on. Find out if the area is prone to flooding, tornadoes, or other extreme weather hazards. Discover whether the dirt road washes out in winter or if you're likely to get snowed in. Consider the prevailing winds in your weather calculations, too. It's great to have some kind of windbreaks (hills, trees, or both) that naturally obstruct storms and high winds. If the property has deciduous trees, try to scope it out in winter; when the leaves are gone, you'll get a much better view of the land.

THE OUTSIDE WORLD If you're getting older or if you have some sort of health-related issue, you may not want to live too terribly far away from a hospital, or at least a small medical facility. This modern asset can be a life saver (no pun intended). Other useful elements of contemporary living can include things such as schools (if you have any children), shopping, gas stations, and restaurants. You're probably thinking: "Restaurants? But we're going to eat all of our own food that we grow or hunt!" That's a fine goal, but here's the reality check: If you spend one too many days eating nothing but moose meat, you'll end up mounting your own head over the fire place. Trust us—you're going to need a restaurant within a few hours' drive of your homestead. So here's your homework question. How self-sufficient can you really be (especially long-term), and what can you not live without (literally and figuratively)?

BUG-OUT COMPATIBLE Perhaps you're one of those people who wants a piece of land for an emergency stronghold (also known as a bug-out location). A bug-out friendly property should have great resources, such as potable water, wood, wild edible plants, and lots of game animals. The piece of property shouldn't be so far away that you couldn't reach it on foot during a crisis. If you're not living there and working from the site, about a three- or four-day walk from your home or workplace is pushing the limits. Finally, the property should also be defensible by its occupants, just in case things get really rough for a while.

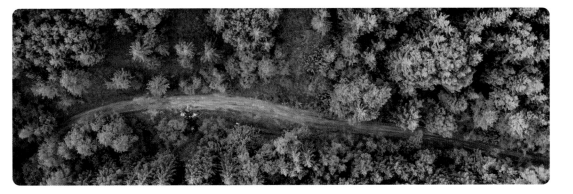

99 RUN ON SUNLIGHT

During an emergency or disaster it's common to lose power for extended periods of time—sometimes even weeks. Considering how often we rely on portable devices, a small solar generator allows you to keep using your critical devices long past spare battery packs have died.

The Goal Zero Yeti series of portable generators are widely recommended. Not only can they charge using a variety of fixed and portable solar panels, they will also charge from AC wall power, along with 12-volt power from most vehicles and vessels. This generator system has an easy-to-use, informative display and replaceable batteries. It is also chainable to other batteries, so the main unit can extend its capacity. It has five to 10 different output ports (depending on model), to provide a variety of power options for 12 volt, USB, and AC. You won't need fuel to operate it (thus making it safe to use indoors), and it's silent since it does not use a noisy internal combustion system to generate power.

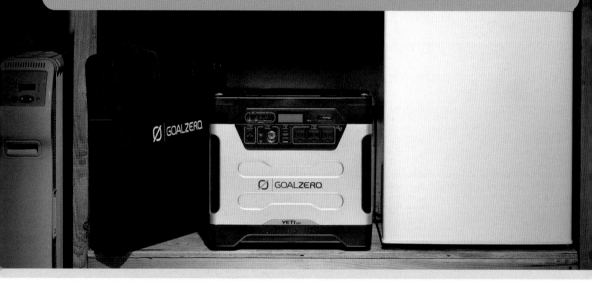

100 GET POWER IN YOUR POCKET

When you're on the move, you might not be able to bring a larger power supply or charging system with you. Under those circumstances, you will need a portable solution that can be stored in your go bag.

Depending on your individual situation and needs, this handy device might even be considered useful as an everyday carry item—for instance, if you're spending a lot of time in the field away from opportunities to charge your electronics.

Additionally, a portable charger can be useful for when you go camping, hiking, or do other outdoor recreational activities.

Solar chargers that have carabiners or mounting straps are easily attached to your backpack or go bag so that it can work in daylight while you go about your business. You also want to have multiple USB ports, the ability to also charge from AC power, good-quality battery cells and solar panels, and a fuel gauge to show how much power is left in reserve. Some models also have built-in fault indicators, and flashlights run by the unit's internal power.

Pocket models aren't much bigger than a tube of lipstick and can carry enough power for a full charge on a mobile phone (depending on your model). Just remember to keep it fully charged so that, when you need it, there will be power aplenty to charge your devices.

101 BACK UP YOUR PLANS

While not a long-term solution for the loss of the power grid, this DIY battery system can charge critical electronic devices to give you more than a week's worth of use. Sometimes, just having access to a limited yet reliable power supply can make a big difference.

If you want to use this system indoors, use an absorbed glass mat (AGM) battery; the traditional lead-acid types can produce harmful fumes. You can purchase a 55 AH (ampere-hour) 12-volt battery from home-improvement or boating stores, or repurpose one from a boat, RV, or other vehicle. You can order batteries with even more capacity, but size and cost will both increase. You will also need a battery wall charger, a cigarette lighter adapter, a cell phone car charger, and a voltmeter to test the setup.

Wear safety goggles and take great care when working with batteries. AGM batteries are less toxic than lead-acid car batteries but still contain acid.

STEP 1 Using the voltmeter, ensure that your battery is fully charged. If you store your battery, check up on it every three months. If the charge drops below 12.4 volts, charge it so it'll be ready to go when the lights go out. A smart charger with an automatic trickle charge mode will keep the battery fully charged for when you need it.

STEP 2 Attach the cigarette lighter port to your battery. It's easy—the port attaches to wires with a set of jumper cable-like alligator clips.

STEP 3 Plug in the phone charger, as you would in your car, and charge up your phone. Your results will vary based on the number and capacity of the devices that you're charging, and the total capacity of the battery, but modern smartphones will recharge about 25 times with your typical fully charged car battery—more so for those larger-capacity marine batteries.

STEP 4 Periodically insert the voltmeter into the cigarette lighter adapter to check on your voltage—you don't want to run your battery down too far. As when it's in storage, never let it drop below 12.4 volts.

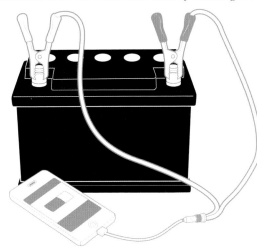

102 UNDERSTAND BATTERY CAPACITY

The milliampere-hour, abbreviated to mAH, is a unit of electrical charge frequently used to rate the capacity of batteries. In order to understand how large a battery you need to charge one or more of your devices, add up each device's battery mAH and compare it to the battery that you are using to charge them. You'll have a good approximation of how many charges you have left in your battery before needing to recharge. Ideally, you'll want a battery that fully charges the intended device to at least 80% or better. For those looking at large batteries, 1 AH = 1000 mAH.

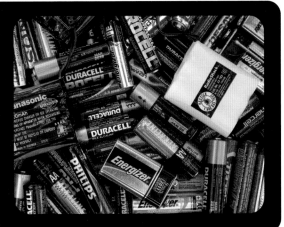

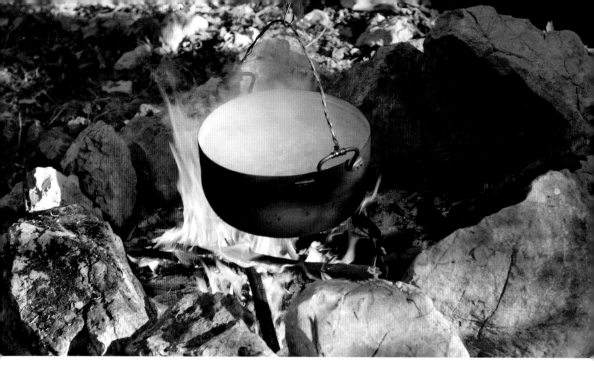

103   KEEP YOUR WATER CLEAN

If you have used up all of your stored water and there are no other reliable clean-water sources, it may become necessary to treat any unknown water source to make it potable. Treat all water, no matter what you plan on using it for. Besides potentially having a bad odor and taste, contaminated water can contain microorganisms as well as other contaminants.

There are several ways to treat water, but none of them are perfect, so if time and resources allow, the best practice is to combine methods. Before treating, filter out debris and other particulates by using cheesecloth, coffee filters, or available clean cloth.

USE ULTRAVIOLET The ultraviolet (UV) light water treatment is fast and easy, and you can use a special UV light device (see item 244) or sunlight. To treat up to 33 ounces (1 liter) at a time, just stir the device for 90 seconds in the water and it's ready for you to drink.

BOIL IT This is the safest method of treating water, achieved by simply bringing water to a rolling boil for 5 minutes. The water will taste better if you aerate it by pouring the water back and forth between two clean containers.

TRY CHLORINE Use only regular household liquid bleach containing 5.25 to 6.0 percent sodium hypochlorite. Do not use bleach that is scented, color safe, or has added cleansers. Use a newly opened or unopened bottle, as the potency of bleach diminishes with time. Add 8 drops of bleach for each gallon (4 liters) of water, stir, and let stand for 30 minutes. The water should have a slight bleach odor. If not, repeat the dosage and let stand another 15 minutes. If it still does not smell of chlorine, discard it and find another source of water.

DISTILL IT Distillation has the advantage of removing other contaminants besides microbes but unfortunately is also the most complicated method of treating water unless you own a distiller unit (which may not work if power is unavailable).

METHOD	KILLS MICROBES	REMOVES OTHER CONTAMINANTS*
UV LIGHT		No
BOILING	Yes	No
CHLORINATION	Yes	
DISTILLATION		Yes

* HEAVY METALS, SALTS, AND OTHER CHEMICALS

104 TRY SOLAR DISINFECTION

If you have a clear glass or plastic bottle, some water, and a sunny day, you can harness the power of the sun's light to make your water much safer to drink. Largely advocated for developing countries, solar water disinfection is also useful in any post-disaster circumstance anywhere in the world, although it's best applied in equatorial countries that can provide abundant strong sunlight.

The most common solar disinfection technique is to expose a clear plastic bottle full of questionable water to the sun for a minimum of one full day. The sun's natural UV light kills or damages almost all biological contaminants in the water. This method is easy to do, it's essentially free, and it offers good (but not complete) bacterial and viral disinfection.

Use only clear bottles that are 66 ounces (2 liters) or smaller in size for effective treatment. The water must be clear, so filter it first if necessary. Set the water bottle out in direct sunlight for an entire day, or leave it out for two days if the weather is overcast.

There are some challenges, though: This method is not effective in rainy weather. It offers no residual disinfection and is not as effective against bacterial spores and cyst stages of some parasites. It's not 100 percent effective, but it's better than taking your chances with untreated water.

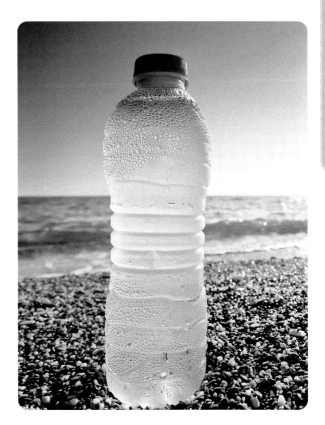

105 DISTILL WATER PROPERLY

Distillation is simple in principle, involving boiling water and then collecting the vapor that condenses. If you lack special lab equipment or a commercial distiller, you can improvise using a large pot, some paracord, and a mug.

STEP 1 Fill the pot halfway with water.

STEP 2 Tie the cup to the handle on the pot's lid so that the cup will hang right side up while the lid is upside down. Check to be sure that, when you lower the lid, the cup is not dangling into the water. If possible, add some ice to the inverted lid to speed up condensation below.

STEP 3 Boil the water for 20 minutes.

STEP 4 Carefully lift the lid. The water that has dripped from the lid into the cup is distilled and safe to drink.

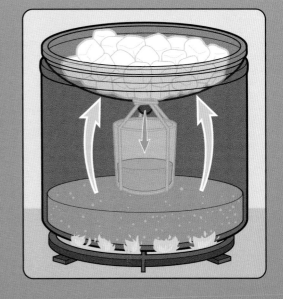

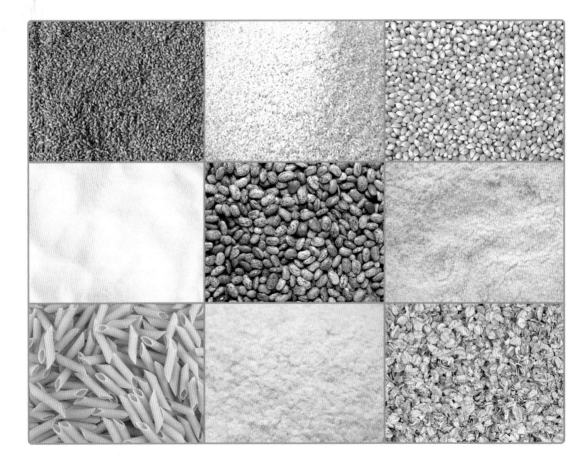

Dry goods and a few other foods can be safely stored for years in a variety of containers, when packaged along with the appropriate desiccant or oxygen absorbing materials. One popular combination is a five-gallon (19 l) food grade bucket lined with a thick Mylar food storage bag. Place the bag inside the bucket, fill this bag nearly full of dry food, add the right amount of oxygen absorbing packets and heat seal the bag closed (with a special tool or a flat iron for hair care). The oxygen absorber product will actually draw a vacuum on the bag over the next few days, and as long as the vacuum holds (the bag looks "sucked in"), the dry goods should last for decades. Place the lid on the bucket and store it in a cool, dark, dry place. Depending on the contents, each gallon bucket should feed one person for 3-4 weeks. When packing your food, you can set up each bucket to hold a large volume of one type of food (the easiest way), or you can do smaller Mylar bags for rationing purposes and combined product

buckets. You don't need the O2 absorbers in everything. Sugar, honey and salt will never need them; but grain, powdered milk, and most other foods should include them. 100CC oxygen absorber packets are a great choice for smaller containers, as you can parcel out the right amount of product for different jar and bag sizes. You'll need 1—100CC packet for a 1 quart (1 l) canning jar, and 4—100 CC packets for 1 gallon (4 l)jars and containers. 5 gallon (19 l) buckets of food usually take the equivalent of 1500 to 2000 CCs of product. Desiccant packs (different from oxygen absorber packets) may also be placed in foods that have some residual moisture, like dried fruit and jerky, but these are not suitable foods for 30-year storage.

107 PLAN FOR THE LONG HAUL

Certain foods, if properly stored, can last 30 years or more in your pantry. Remember, do not try these long-term storage methods with even very slightly moist foods, to avoid the risk of botulism. Not sure if a foodstuff is dry enough? Place it on a piece of paper and whack it with a hammer. If it shatters, it's dry. If it squishes, it definitely isn't. And if it breaks but leaves a little spot of water or oil, it's still too moist. Err on the side of safety—your family's life is literally on the line.

STORE FOR UP TO 30 YEARS
Wheat · White rice · Dried corn · White sugar · Pinto beans · Rolled oats · Dry pasta · Potato flakes · Salt · Nonfat powdered milk

NOT SUITABLE FOR LONG-TERM STORAGE
Dried fruit · Pearled barley · Jerky · Nuts · Peanuts & oily seeds · Dried eggs · Brown rice · Whole-wheat flour · Milled grain · Brown sugar

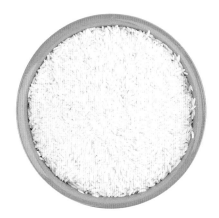

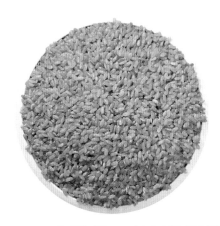

108 DON'T FORGET FIFO

A basic rule of any food pantry is "First In, First Out." What that means: Keep track of the expiration dates on items, and swap them out as they approach culinary old age. That bagged rice is good for a year? After 11 months, replace it with a new bag and enjoy a nice jambalaya. You should never have to throw anything away, just keep using ingredients and replacing them as needed. That way, if and when disaster does strike, dinner's not going to be expired okra served over bug-infested rice.

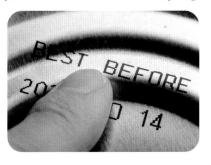

109 COUNT CALORIES

We're accustomed to reading food labels to make sure they don't have too many calories, too much fat, or too many carbs. In a short-term emergency, you turn this wisdom on its head. Your body needs fuel, and fat and sugar are the fastest ways to fuel up. Your go-bag and short-term food stashes should include things like protein bars, MREs, peanut butter, jelly, crackers, and other calorie-dense, easy-to-eat items. That doesn't mean your best survival foods are pork rinds and soda pop—you should strive for some nutritional value, which is why nutrition bars are a good, reasonably priced staple.

GROW YOUR OWN MEDICINE CHEST

Even with limited space, you can grow your own herbal remedies. These won't replace proper medical care, but they're nice to have on hand in a pinch—or a bruise.

Ⓐ **ALOE VERA** Very soothing to burns and scalds, this tender plant is best grown in a container so that it can be brought inside for the winter (unless you live in a tropical climate).

Ⓑ **BORAGE** The flowers can be soaked in alcohol to make a mood-boosting tonic.

Ⓒ **PEPPERMINT** Similar to pennyroyal, peppermint can be a great tonic for digestion. Fresh peppermint, though, along with pennyroyal and other strong mints, should not be consumed by women who are (or may be) pregnant, as food or drinks that contain fresh, strong mint leaves can be dangerous to the baby.

Ⓓ **COMFREY** The cooked, mashed roots of comfrey are used for a topical treatment for arthritis, bruises, burns, and sprains. Just don't eat it. Recent research shows that it is damaging to the liver if eaten in quantity.

Ⓔ **YARROW** Crushed yarrow leaves and flowers can be placed on cuts and scratches in order to stop bleeding and reduce the chance of infection.

Ⓕ **LEMON BALM** This plant makes an outstanding topical agent for cold sores, and it is often used as a calming "nightcap" tea to fight insomnia.

Ⓖ **ECHINACEA** This perennial wildflower is used in preparations to protect against colds and flu, minor infections, and a host of other ailments while boosting the immune system.

Ⓗ **PENNYROYAL** This great-smelling mint relative can be crushed and applied to the skin as a very effective bug repellent. The leaves can also be crushed and then applied to wounds as an antiseptic, or brewed as a tea to settle upset stomachs.

Ⓘ **LAVENDER** Typically used as a fragrance today, lavender has been used since ancient times to treat bug bites, burns, and skin disorders, and to relieve itching and rashes and reduce swelling. It should not be used by pregnant or nursing women, or small children.

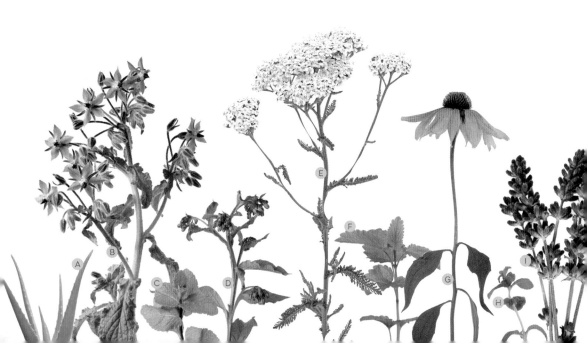

111 MAKE A SELF-WATERING CONTAINER GARDEN

Containers are a great way to grow food in small spaces or to add extra growing space in and around your home and property. Many vegetables grow well in containers. It's best to use a self-watering container—this reduces your labor and also allows plants to suck up the water they need through their roots, which can help to eliminate any over- or under-watering. Daily watering can be annoying, and commercial self-watering containers can be pricey. Here's how to make your own, with some simple-to-obtain supplies. You'll need two 5-gallon (19-l) food containers, an 8-ounce (225-g) plastic deli container of the sort you'd buy potato salad in, a length of plastic pipe, and a power drill.

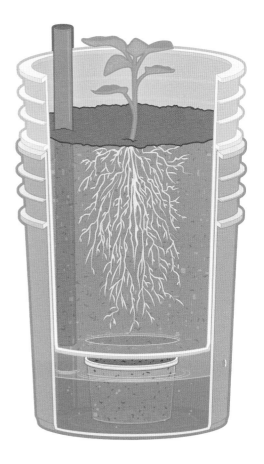

STEP 1 Drill some small holes all the way around the deli container, spaced about an inch (2.5 cm) apart.

STEP 2 Using a 3-inch (8-cm) hole saw, make a hole in the bottom of one of your large containers, and then follow up with smaller drainage holes all around the central hole. Then, using a 1¼-inch (3-cm) hole saw, drill a water hole for the pipe to run through.

STEP 3 Assemble the container, placing the plastic deli container in the bottom tub (the one without the holes) and the drilled-out tub on top of it.

STEP 4 Determine where the inner container's bottom is (holding the whole container up to a strong light should make this apparent). Drill a small overflow hole about a quarter inch (0.6 cm) below the inner tub's bottom.

STEP 5 Run the watering pipe down through the 1¼-inch (3-cm) hole.

STEP 6 Fill the container with potting soil (it will fill the deli container as well) and plant your produce.

STEP 7 Pour water down the pipe until it flows out the drainage hole. This will now water your plants through their roots. Every week or so, pour a little water down the pipe and see how your reservoir is doing.

112 WATCH THE PETS

There are a whole host of things you should take into consideration when planning a survival garden. First and foremost are ease of planting, yield of crops, and nutritional density. You want to grow as much as you can as easily as possible. And you want those crops to be nutritious. You also want them to be safe for all members of your household—including Fido and Fluffy. Stay informed about which plants to keep out of reach of your pets. Aloe, garlic, leeks, rhubarb, and certain kinds of holly can be toxic to both dogs and cats if ingested. Effects can range from nausea (indicated by drooling) to tremors and death. Check with your veterinarian if you have any questions.

STOCK YOUR TOOL SHED

No matter what advertisers may want you to believe, there's no one tool that will get you out of every jam. But if you stock up on these essentials, you'll be well set to face a multitude of issues.

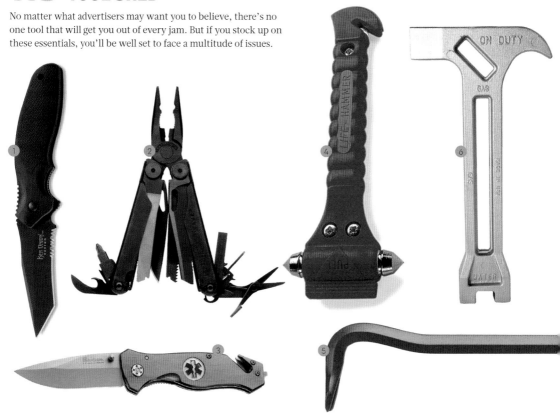

1 TACTICAL KNIFE While hopefully you won't have to protect yourself from attackers, it could happen, and there's no harm in having a good self-defense knife just in case. This sort of knife is sometimes used as a backup to firearms by those in the military and law enforcement. They're rugged and relatively large, with a razor-sharp blade.

2 MULTITOOL The versatile multitool got its start as the venerable Swiss Army knife and has a wide number of fold-out tools including screwdrivers, pliers, saws, and knife blades. Though it's not as effective as a fully stocked toolbox, it's a great deal easier to carry with you.

3 RESCUE KNIFE Also known as an EMS knife, this handy tool is commonly carried by all manner of emergency services personnel, from firefighters to police to paramedics. It's a folding knife with a blade that's at least partly serrated and features two very important accessories: a seat-belt cutter and a window breaker. If you don't wear it on your belt, keep one in your car.

4 RESCUE TOOL If you prefer not to keep a knife in your car, then this rescue tool can help you escape from your own vehicle after an accident as well as allowing you to help free others who may be in peril. It's designed to be mounted inside your vehicle for easy access, and it will break side and rear windows easily and cut seat belts safely.

5 CROW BAR This is the epitome of a tool that you may not use all that often but you will be glad to have one when you need it. In disasters they are primarily used for forcing locks, doors and windows open after being damaged, as well as for various secondary uses such as clearing debris, prying apart boards, removing nails, and even self-defense.

6 UTILITY SHUT-OFF TOOL While you can use regular household tools to shut off your utilities in a pinch, having a

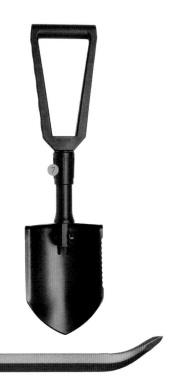

114 FILL YOUR HOUSEHOLD TOOL KIT

Even if you're not the handy type who likes to fix things, you should still consider having a basic hand tool kit in your home. It's better to have a tool and never use it than need a tool and not have it. During a disaster or in an emergency you may not have the ability to go buy tools, so having a kit handy becomes an extension of your emergency kit. And who knows, you might also be able to fix something with the tools now that you have them. Household tool kits are often sold in complete packages with a storage case. A good general tool kit includes the following.

- Hammer/mallet
- Saw
- Screwdrivers (Phillips and flat, in various sizes)
- Razor knife
- Wrenches (adjustable and open end, in various sizes)
- Hex keys (in various sizes)
- Wire cutter/stripper
- Pliers (slip-joint and groove-joint)
- Needle-nose pliers
- Digital voltmeter
- Tape measure
- Level

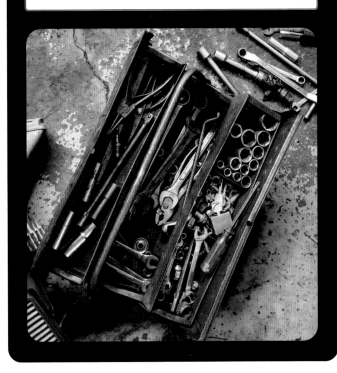

combined tool makes it really easy to grab and go or include in your disaster tool kit. Not only does this non-sparking tool allow you to shut off your gas and water, it can also be used to do some light rescue work, such as prying open doors and breaking windows.

7 FOLDING SHOVEL Also called an entrenching tool, these compact spades were originally designed for military use. However, there are a myriad of civilian uses for disasters, winter, camping, and self-defense. Those that have a serrated edge can also be used as a saw. The ability to dig latrines is of special note in disasters when water is scarce or unavailable.

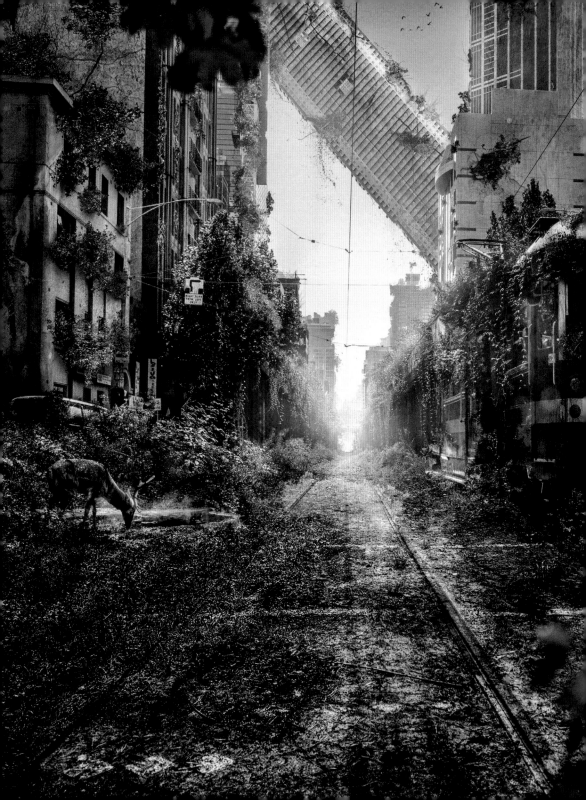

EXTREME OUTCOMES

Being prepared means considering a range of possible outcomes. It's possible that the crisis we feared will turn out to be nothing more than a minor inconvenience. It's also possible that things could go the other way.

For those who want to hope for the best while planning for the worst, we humbly offer this chapter of worst-case scenarios and considerations. While it's highly unlikely that a pandemic will wipe out civilization or destroy our economy, the chance of these extreme outcomes is never zero. And for some of us, knowing what to do in these dystopian circumstances is comforting, even if we hope we'll never have to use this knowledge.

BRACE FOR IMPACT When the worst happens, it's time to assemble your team, identify the worst threats, and create a plan of action to survive those threatening issues. Remember, "teamwork makes the dream work," so choose the right people to surround you.

BUG OUT While we all hope it never comes to this, "bugging out" should always be considered as a back-up plan for survival. Since many different scenarios could make it unsafe to remain in your home, you'll need a plan, supplies, and a preselected destination to make your exodus successful.

ENDURE THE WORST Tough situations can create tough people. In the event that things should take a turn for the worse, it's important to remain alert to changing threats, stay strong, and bring the things you'll need to start over someplace new.

115 GET READY FOR A FALL

TEOTWAWKI (The End of the World as We Know It) certainly sounds ominous and un-survivable. But if we look back into history, we can see that many "worlds" have ended, only to give rise to a different culture or civilization—not without growing pains, but with plenty of survivors. The fall of Rome, two World Wars, and many other historical events have been game changers, ending some lives and changing the survivors' world. Here are some ways it could happen.

SOCIAL COLLAPSE Sometimes people just can't see eye to eye. Civil wars, religious conflicts, and class wars have taken countless lives over the centuries and affected entire continents. On a smaller scale, race riots, gang wars, and rioting have immobilized entire cities. When civility is lost between neighbors, societies have a hard time surviving.

GOVERNMENT COLLAPSE Throughout recorded history, many governments have fallen apart due to a variety of stressors. When a government system fails to be sustainable or fails its people one too many times, leaders can topple.

ECONOMIC COLLAPSE Zimbabwe's economy collapsed in 2008 due to hyperinflation, among other factors. Argentina's economy fell apart a few years before that when the country defaulted on international loans. The world's economic crisis post-pandemic may take years to resolve itself.

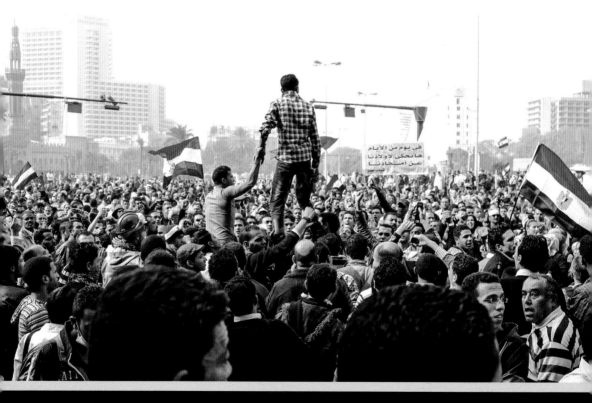

116 STOCK UP FOR THE CRASH

The ideal lifestyle after a currency collapse is one that doesn't require money. But few folks today have the skills and the land to be completely self-reliant. In the event that a currency fails, bartering goods and services can fill the void until a new monetary system is established. So you'll want to be the one with the possessions and skill sets that would be valuable in a time without money. You'll also want to conceal the location of these things — and guard them with your life.

117 BUILD A TEAM

In the crime-ridden aftermath of a collapse, being surrounded by like-minded individuals with complementary skills could be your best plan of action.

Living in close proximity to each other could offer great advantages to all of you. Try to make friends with folks who bring these skill sets to the table.

- Military and law-enforcement backgrounds
- Medical and dental skills
- Food production experience
- Vehicle repair experience
- Building and fabricating skills
- Firefighting background

118 UNDERSTAND THE REAL THREAT

The two biggest threats during a social, government, or economic collapse are violence and an inability to provide for your basic needs. The issue of violent crime is by far the most dangerous by-product of unrest and an ever-present reality during instances of community meltdown. The rates of murder, theft, arson, rape, and home invasion have always increased in these scenarios. Regardless of the type of collapse, take the steps to protect yourself, your friends, and your family.

HIDE YOUR WEALTH Your wealth may come in the form of money, water, food, ammunition, animals, or any other kind of desired commodity. Don't flaunt it, and don't let anyone outside your circle know what you have or where it is—even before a collapse.

GET ARMED An armed person is a lot more daunting to a predator. Knives, machetes, axes, or even a baseball bat can help to protect you and yours.

GET TRAINING A tool for self-defense is good, but the training to go with it is great. Find a local business that offers self-defense training with different weapons. Train regularly, and make sure that your family members have some skills as well. You can even take lessons from former police officers for a stiff dose of reality and an insight into the criminal minds they have faced.

HAVE A PLAN Devising plans within plans may keep you up a little longer at night, but isn't that better than going to sleep with your head in the sand? Believe in the old adage, "Failing to plan is planning to fail."

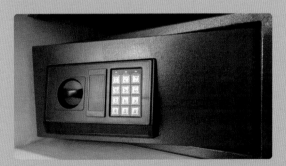

119 HAIL THE NEW CHIEF

A government collapsing on its own is a fairly rare event in history. More often, you see piecemeal changes occur over time. Unless you're planning to take the throne yourself, the best advice during a government collapse is to get as far away as possible. It may take years for a stable society to emerge from the chaos after coups, assassinations, invasions, and the like. If you cannot flee, or refuse to become a refugee, you'd better get on board with your new leadership if you wish to survive.

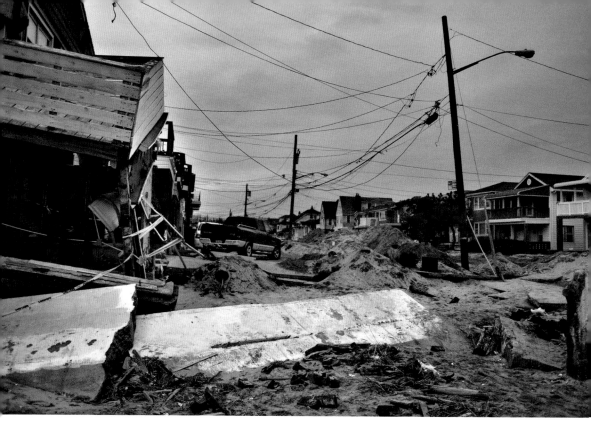

120 DECIDE WHETHER TO STAY

Whether to stay put or bug out could be the toughest and most important decision you make in times of disaster. While much writing about survival focuses on bugging out, in reality many situations are best ridden out in a secure, well-provisioned home or place of business. How do you know what to do when things are scary? Here are a few things to consider when you're trying to decide if it's better to shelter in place or to get out of Dodge.

The authorities announce that your area should evacuate	The situation is worsening, and you decide that travel is safer than staying put	You have a bug-out location prepared for this situation	You have the necessary gear and skills to survive wherever you may go	You are meeting up with trusted allies who are better prepared and equipped	BUG OUT!
The authorities announce that you should shelter in place	The situation is not safe to travel through	You don't have a functional vehicle	You don't have the gear and skills to survive in the outdoors	You have nowhere else to go	STAY PUT

121 GRAB YOUR GO BAG

A go bag is a collection of items that you would need to survive if you had to flee your home with no guarantee of shelter, food, or water during an emergency. Think of it as your survival insurance policy. There may not be one universally agreed-upon set of equipment but, with a good core set of items, you can put together a go bag suited for a wide variety of situations.

It's best to use a backpack so that you can easily carry your gear. Fill it up with the minimum following things, with items sealed in zip-top bags to keep them organized and prevent them getting wet.

- Shelter items like a small tent and sleeping bag (if you want to go ultraminimalist, pack a tarp and a space blanket)
- Drinking water and purification equipment
- High-calorie, no-cook foods such as protein bars, peanut butter, trail mix, etc.
- First-aid, sanitation, and hygiene supplies
- Several fire-starting options
- A small pot for boiling water or cooking
- Basic tools such as a knife, duct tape, and paracord
- Extra clothes appropriate for all seasons
- Flashlight with extra batteries
- Cash and a spare debit card
- A thumb drive with a backup of important documents: bank info, insurance documents, wills, and personal items such as family photos or videos

Stash your main go bag safe and ready to go in a secure location, with smaller versions in your car and office. It's also a good idea for you to have everyday carry (EDC) items—survival essentials that you can carry in your pocket or purse.

HOME GO BAG

Emergency rations (MREs, food bars, etc) · Bottled water · Tent & tarp · Sleeping bag · Space blanket · Change of rugged clothes · Flashlight & extra batteries · Pocket knife · Can opener · Heavy cord · Battery- or crank-operated weather and AM/FM radio · First aid kit · Sanitation kit · Medications & extra eyeglasses, hearing aid batteries, etc. · Whistle · Change of shoes & socks · Duct tape · Razor blades · Water filter · Water purification tablets · Solar charger · Battery pack · Crow bar · Utility shutoff tool · Fishing kit · Folding shovel · Reflective traffic vest · Lantern · Work gloves · Lighter or fire-starting kit

CAR GO BAG

Emergency rations (MREs, food bars, etc.) · Bottled water · Tent & tarp · Space blanket · Change of rugged clothes · Flashlight & extra batteries · Pocket knife · Can opener · Heavy cord · First-aid kit · Whistle · Change of shoes & socks · Duct tape · Razor blades · Water filter · Water purification tablets · Fishing kit · Folding shovel · Snow chains & a bag of sand · Jumper cables, flares, tow strap · Reflective traffic vest · Work gloves · Lighter or fire-starting kit

OFFICE GO BAG

Emergency rations (MREs, food bars, etc.) · Bottled water · Space blanket · Flashlight & extra batteries · Whistle · Change of shoes & socks · Reflective traffic vest

COMPACT EDC GO BAG

Flashlight & extra batteries · Pocket knife · Whistle · Battery pack · Lighter or fire-starting kit

123 AVOID OVERLOAD

Maybe you were in the military and you survived brutal forced marches with a 100 pound (45-kg) pack on your back, or a scout leader made you hike up a mountain carrying half your body weight. Maybe you never backpacked before in your life. All these scenarios have the same factor: a body can only carry so much weight so far before falling to the ground. We must keep limitations in mind when we start loading up a go bag, for good reason. If you're bugging out, you are in a tough situation. You'll be stressed and maybe underfed or unrested. This diminishes your load bearing abilities. You may also need to run with the pack or swim. That heavy rucksack will stop these activities. Keep the weight as low as you can, while still carrying the essentials. Otherwise, the bag becomes an anchor.

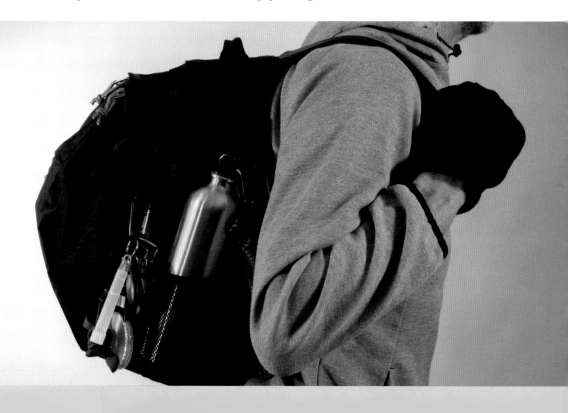

125 HIT THE ROAD QUICKLY

In some situations, you don't need a full go-bag. You just require enough to get out of Dodge. This kit (aka, your "Get Home Bag") is much leaner and meaner than the average go-bag, and its purpose is clear: getting you home. If you are planning on camping out at your house, not camping out in the woods, this is your go-to. Have one in your car and one at the office. Find ways to modify the bug out bag list to make the kit smaller, lighter, and cheaper (just in case it gets stolen out of your car or at work). Shelter could be just a tarp and fleece blanket or a space blanket if funds or storage room are limited. The water can just be bottles from a store and disinfection tablets so you can refill your two bottles as you go. Remember, this kit is just to keep you safe until you reach your real gear at home.

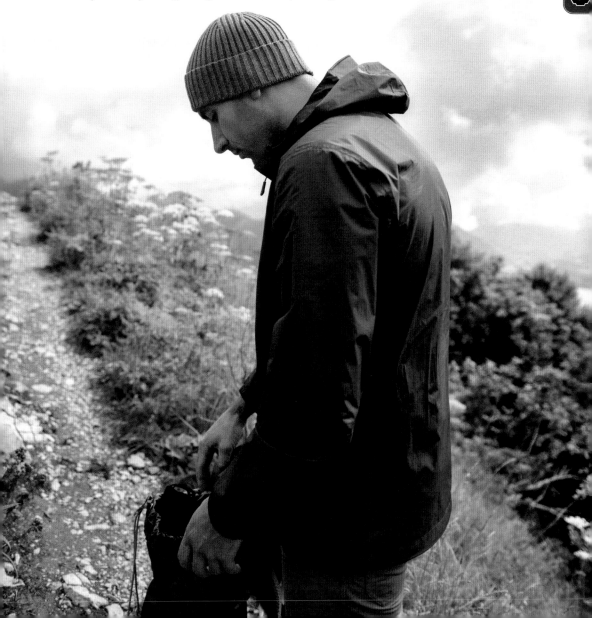

126 WATCH OUT FOR BAD GUYS

Tough times can bring out the best in people—but they can also bring bad guys out of the woodwork. There's a certain sort of sociopath who lives to wield power over others. These folks often appear charismatic, smart, and competent at first. Don't jump to conclusions, but don't be misled either. Here are some traits to watch out for before throwing your support behind that charismatic newcomer.

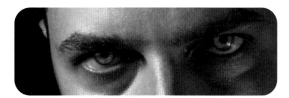

CHARMING Sociopaths are often incredibly charming, seeming like born leaders. In fact, they are excellent con artists, using charm to manipulate and control others.

ENTITLED Sociopaths believe that they are better than others and will stop at nothing to prevail, as they genuinely believe they deserve it.

LACK EMPATHY Sociopaths can be nice and helpful when they need to, but they lack true, deep emotions. Similarly, they show no remorse for their actions. If you get an apology from a sociopath, it's because he or she wants something from you. They have few or no real friends or relationships.

BLAME OTHERS Nobody likes to mess up, but most folks will admit error and move on. The true sociopath always manages to pin the blame on someone else. They can often be bullies, intimidating or manipulating people to get what they want—or just for fun.

127 SET UP A BUG-OUT VEHICLE

If you have to bug out, you're not having a good day. This is not some glorious movie scene where you drive your doomsday wagon down the road bathed in looks of shock and awe from bystanders. Bugging out means fleeing for your life. Now that the fantasy has been dispelled, let's have a real discussion about the things that would help you in an actual bug out vehicle.

CARGO ROOM Your supplies are your lifeline. They are also bulky and heavy, but they're worth every bit of weight and space. This makes cargo capacity a major factor.

4X4 All-wheel drive or a 4x4 option could mean the difference between getting out and getting stuck.

GROUND CLEARANCE You don't need a monster truck, but you don't need a low sports car either.

PASSENGER ROOM You should have enough room for your family or group.

LOW PROFILE One more point to consider is blending in. If your vehicle has tools and cargo strapped all over it, others may be interested in the provisions you clearly have. Instead, maybe you should be driving something that looks like a work vehicle or a soccer mom mobile. You could still have all the post-apocalypse supplies you want, but this way you're not advertising it to the panicked masses.

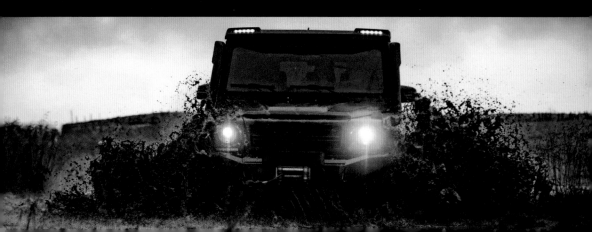

128 KNOW WHERE YOU'RE GOING

Bugging out without a destination makes you a refugee. If you have an off-the-grid property that you have been developing into a homestead, you already have a great BOL (bug out location). But what if you don't, or if you had to leave that self-sufficient property? Consider a "Site B" as a back-up plan. Your back-up site could be virtually anything and virtually anywhere (as long as you can get to it in a crisis). Site B could be a cabin in the wilds, or the abandoned farm your family once worked in the middle of nowhere. It could be the undeveloped land of a friend or family member or even a spot that you picked on land you don't own. The site needs to have water and natural resources, be off the beaten path and defensible, and it should have a hidden cache of supplies.

129 START OVER

If you want to know what life would be like in a post-disaster, bug-out setting, go live with some homeless folks for a while in a rough part of the world. Living in tents and constantly being victimized by other people is pretty much what that life is all about. You don't dare set up a camp and leave it unattended for long. You could return from a food run to find every last item stolen, or just destroyed out of spite. And you can forget about a good night's sleep:. That's why it's so vital to bug out as a group, so you can post watches and take care of each other. And that is also why you should choose a remote place away from hostile strangers.

DON'T GO ALONE Bugging out alone is a recipe for trouble. You need help, various skills, and more gear than you can possibly carry in a real bug-out situation. It may seem like a badass character type, the lone wolf survivor is a figment of Hollywood's imagination. Lone wolves seldom live very long cut off from all other people. After all, throughout history the worst punishment a community could give was exile, being forced to live out on your own.

PREPARE TO START OVER How do you put your life back together after a bug-out-worthy disaster? Very few people in modern times have had to bug out and then start their life over again. You need money, documentation of your identity, and a place to go. You may be scrambling to find a new place to live. You may also need a new source of income as your money quickly runs out. In localized crisis situations, aid often floods in from other areas—but it's an uncharted territory to rebuild your life in the wake of mass destruction and casualties. Let's just hope we never have to find out how hard it could be to start all over again.

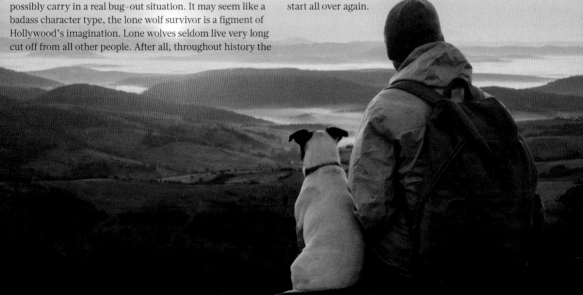

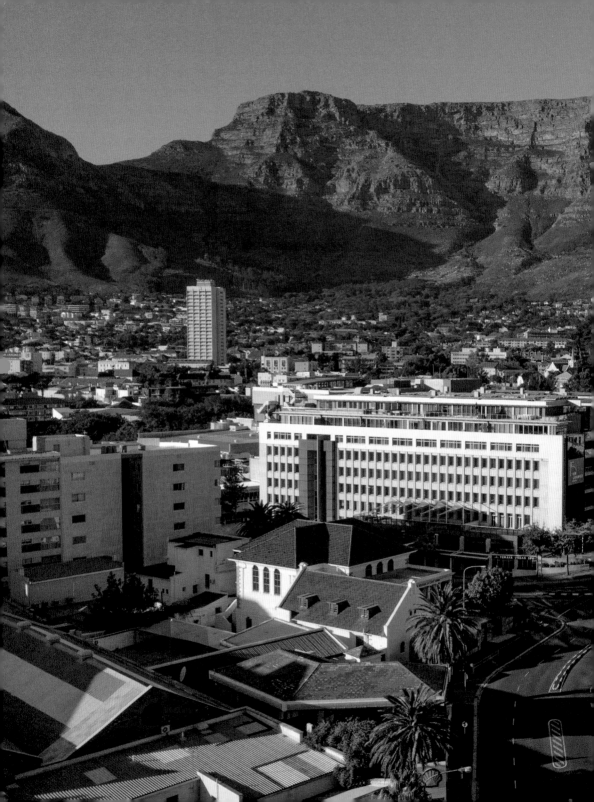

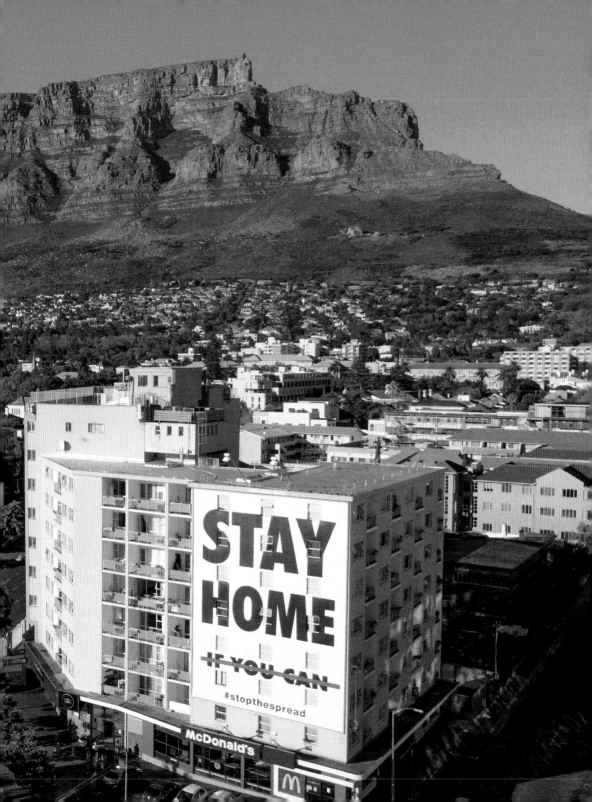

130 COORDINATE AND EVACUATE FORMS

When disaster strikes, it's important to have a plan for where to go, whom to call, and how to meet up. This form makes it easy for everyone to know the details.

FAMILY CONTACTS LIST

FAMILY'S LAST NAME: _____

STREET ADDRESS: _____

CITY AND STATE: _____ **LAND LINE:** _____

EVERYONE WHO LIVES AT THIS ADDRESS

NAME: _____ **CELL PHONE:** _____ **SPECIAL NEEDS:** _____

EMAIL: _____ **WORK PHONE:** _____ _____

NAME: _____ **CELL PHONE:** _____ **SPECIAL NEEDS:** _____

EMAIL: _____ **WORK PHONE:** _____ _____

NAME: _____ **CELL PHONE:** _____ **SPECIAL NEEDS:** _____

EMAIL: _____ **WORK PHONE:** _____ _____

NAME: _____ **CELL PHONE:** _____ **SPECIAL NEEDS:** _____

EMAIL: _____ **WORK PHONE:** _____ _____

NAME: _____ **CELL PHONE:** _____ **SPECIAL NEEDS:** _____

EMAIL: _____ **WORK PHONE:** _____ _____

NAME: _____ **CELL PHONE:** _____ **SPECIAL NEEDS:** _____

EMAIL: _____ **WORK PHONE:** _____ _____

HOUSEHOLD EVACUATION PLAN

PETS

NAME: _____ BREED: _____ COLOR: _____ MICROCHIP#: _____

NAME: _____ BREED: _____ COLOR: _____ MICROCHIP#: _____

NAME: _____ BREED: _____ COLOR: _____ MICROCHIP#: _____

IF WE'RE SEPARATED DURING AN EMERGENCY, WHAT'S OUR MUSTER POINT NEAR HOME? _____

_____

IF WE CAN'T RETURN HOME, OR ARE TOLD TO EVACUATE, WHAT'S OUR MEETING POINT OUTSIDE THE NEIGHBORHOOD?

_____

WHAT'S OUR ROUTE TO GET THERE? _____

_____

WHAT'S OUR ALTERNATIVE ROUTE IF THE FIRST ONE IS AFFECTED OR ELIMINATED BY DISASTER? _____

_____

IF FAMILY MEMBERS CAN'T REACH ONE ANOTHER, WHO'S OUR OUT-OF-AREA CONTACT PERSON?

NAME: _____ ADDRESS: _____

EMAIL: _____ CELL/HOME/WORK PHONE: _____

131 KNOW WHAT'S SAFE TO EAT

The grocery-store shelves are almost empty, or you just aren't up for venturing out. Maybe there's a power outage on top of it all. What's safe to eat in these tough times?

FOOD IN REFRIGERATOR

HELD ABOVE 40 °F (4 °C) FOR MORE THAN 2 HOURS

Meat, poultry, or seafood (raw, leftover, or thawing; also includes soy meat substitutes, salads, lunch meats, pizza, cans that have been opened, and sauces with fish or meat)	**DISCARD**
Any soft, shredded, or low-fat cheeses	**DISCARD**
Hard cheeses such as cheddar, colby, swiss, parmesan, provolone, romano, or hard cheeses grated in can or jar	**SAFE**
Milk, cream, sour cream, buttermilk, evaporated milk, yogurt, eggnog, soy milk, or opened baby formula	**DISCARD**
Butter, margarine	**SAFE**
All eggs and egg-based products, such as puddings	**DISCARD**
Fresh fruits, if cut up	**DISCARD**
Pre-cut, pre-washed, and/or cooked vegetables, tofu, opened vegetable juice, garlic in oil, or potato salad	**DISCARD**
Opened fruit juices or canned fruits, along with fresh fruits, coconut, dried or candied fruits, and dates	**SAFE**
Vegetable or cream-based sauces, jam, opened mayonnaise, tartar sauce, and horseradish	**DISCARD*** ** if above 50 °F (10 °C) for over 8 hours*
Soy, barbecue, and taco sauce, peanut butter, jelly, relish, mustard, catsup, olives, pickles, and vinegar-based dressings	**SAFE**
Opened creamy-base dressings or spaghetti sauce	**DISCARD**
Bread, rolls, cakes, cookies, muffins, quick breads, tortillas, waffles, pancakes, bagels, fruit pies, pastries, grains	**SAFE**
Unbaked dough, cooked pasta, rice, potatoes, pasta salads, fresh pasta, cheesecake, or cream-filled pastries or pies	**DISCARD**
Fresh raw vegetables, mushrooms, herbs, and spices	**SAFE**
Casseroles, soups, and stews	**DISCARD**

FOOD IN FREEZER

FOOD TYPE	STILL CONTAINS ICE CRYSTALS AND FEELS AS COLD AS IF REFRIGERATED	THAWED; HELD ABOVE 40 °F (4 °C) FOR MORE THAN 2 HOURS
Meat, poultry, and seafood	**REFREEZE** (Seafood loses some texture and flavor)	**DISCARD**
Milk and soft or semi-soft cheese	**REFREEZE** (Products may lose some texture)	**DISCARD**
Eggs (out of shell) and egg products	**REFREEZE**	**DISCARD**
Ice cream or frozen yogurt	**DISCARD**	**DISCARD**
Hard and shredded cheeses, casseroles with dairy products, cheesecake	**REFREEZE**	**DISCARD**
Fruits (juices and packaged fruits)	**REFREEZE** (Fruit's texture and flavor will change)	**DISCARD**
Vegetables (juices and packaged vegetables)	**REFREEZE** (Vegetables may lose texture and flavor)	**DISCARD** (If above 40 °F (4 °C) for more than 6 hours)
Breads and pastries (breads, rolls, muffins, and cakes without custard fillings)	**REFREEZE**	**REFREEZE**
Cakes, pies, and pastries with custard or cheese fillings	**REFREEZE**	**DISCARD**
Pie crusts, commercial and homemade bread dough	**REFREEZE** (Some quality loss may occur)	**REFREEZE** (Quality loss will be considerable.)
Casseroles (pasta and rice-based)	**REFREEZE**	**DISCARD**
Flour, cornmeal, nuts, waffles, pancakes, bagels	**REFREEZE**	**REFREEZE**
Frozen meals	**REFREEZE**	**DISCARD**

RECOMMENDED READING

This book is a great start, but it only scratches the surface of essential survival information. If you're like us, your interest in surviving the worst goes far beyond pandemics. After all, the world doesn't stop throwing every other challenge at us just because of a killer virus. There are still tornadoes, hurricanes, muggers, and maybe even zombies. (We're joking. There are no zombies. But we've still thought and written about how to survive them, just in case!

Available in fine bookstores everywhere, assuming they're not on lockdown, and that you're allowed to leave your house! Or from your favorite online booksellers any time.

BY JOSEPH PRED

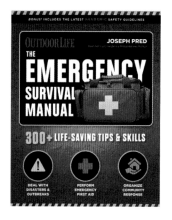

**THE EMERGENCY
SURVIVAL MANUAL**
300+ LIFE-SAVING
TIPS & SKILLS

Over 300 skills for handling disasters of all kinds.

7 x 8.5 paperback
7.5 x 9.5 deluxe flexicover
224 pages

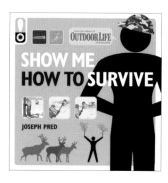

**SHOW ME HOW
TO SURVIVE**
THE HANDBOOK FOR THE
MODERN HERO

Great for kids and young adults, this book is packed with charming and informative illustrations of survival tips.

8 x 8 paperback
144 pages

ALSO AVAILABLE

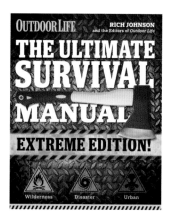

**THE ULTIMATE
SURVIVAL MANUAL**
EXTREME EDITION
By Rich Johnson

Survive everywhere from city streets to outer space.

7 x 8.5 paperback
7.5 x 9.5 deluxe flexicover
256 pages

BY TIM MACWELCH

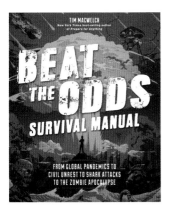

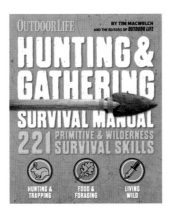

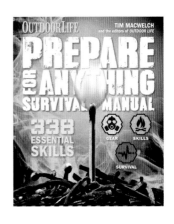

**BEAT THE ODDS
SURVIVAL MANUAL**
FROM GLOBAL PANDEMICS
TO CIVIL UNREST TO
SHARK ATTACKS

Don't take chances with your
life. Read this book.

7.5 x 9.5 deluxe flexicover
224 pages

**HUNTING & GATHERING
SURVIVAL MANUAL**
221 PRIMITIVE & WILDERNESS
SURVIVAL SKILLS

7 x 8.5 paperback
7.5 x 9.5 deluxe flexicover
224 pages

A *New York Times* bestseller

**PREPARE FOR ANYTHING
SURVIVAL MANUAL**
338 ESSENTIAL SKILLS

Keep your family safe.

7 x 8.5 paperback
7.5 x 9.5 deluxe flexicover
240 pages

A *New York Times* bestseller

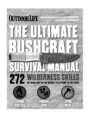

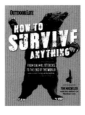

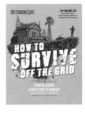

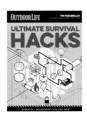

**THE ULTIMATE
BUSHCRAFT
SURVIVAL MANUAL**
272 WILDERNESS
SKILLS

Live off the land
anywhere you go.

7.5 x 9.5 deluxe
flexicover
224 pages

**HOW TO SURVIVE
ANYTHING**
FROM ANIMAL
ATTACKS TO THE END
OF THE WORLD

7 x 8.5 paperback
7.5 x 9.5 deluxe
flexicover
224 pages

A *New York Times*
bestseller

**HOW TO SURVIVE
OFF THE GRID**
FROM BACKYARD
HOMESTEADING
TO BUNKERS

Self-sufficiency guide.

7 x 8.5 paperback
7.5 x 9.5 deluxe
flexicover
224 pages

**ULTIMATE SURVIV-
AL HACKS**
OVER 500 AMAZING
TRICKS THAT
JUST MIGHT SAVE
YOUR LIFE

Packed with DIY tips.

7.5 x 9.5 deluxe
flexicover
224 pages

weldon**owen**

PUBLISHER Roger Shaw
ASSOCIATE PUBLISHER Mariah Bear
SENIOR EDITOR Ian Cannon
CREATIVE DIRECTOR Chrissy Kwasnik
ART DIRECTOR Allister Fein
ILLUSTRATION COORDINATOR
Conor Buckley
MANAGING EDITOR Tarji Rodriguez
PRODUCTION MANAGER Binh Au

© 2020 Weldon Owen International
1150 Brickyard Cove Road
Richmond, CA 94801
www.weldonowen.com

ISBN 978-1-68188-613-8
10 9 8 7 6 5 4 3 2 1
2020 2021 2022 2023
Printed in USA

CREDITS

All photos and illustrations courtesy of Shutterstock
Images, with the following exceptions:

PHOTOS Advil: 38 (C); Banana Boat: 38 (K); FEMA:
70; Goal Zero: 99; George Goslin: 113 (4,6,7);
Jonson & Johnson Consumer Companies, Inc.: 38
(A,B,E,F,N); John Lee: 38 (D,G,M); William Mack:
59; Tim MacWelch: Introduction; Medic Alert
Foundation: 93; Oxy-Sorb: 106; Joseph Pred:
Foreword; RavPower: 100

ILLUSTRATIONS Conor Buckley: 16, 26, 27, 28, 29,
30, 43, 105, 111; Juan Calle: 34; Hayden Foell: 101;
Christine Meighan: 86; Lauren Towner: 56; Carl
Weins: 07; Paul Williams: 41